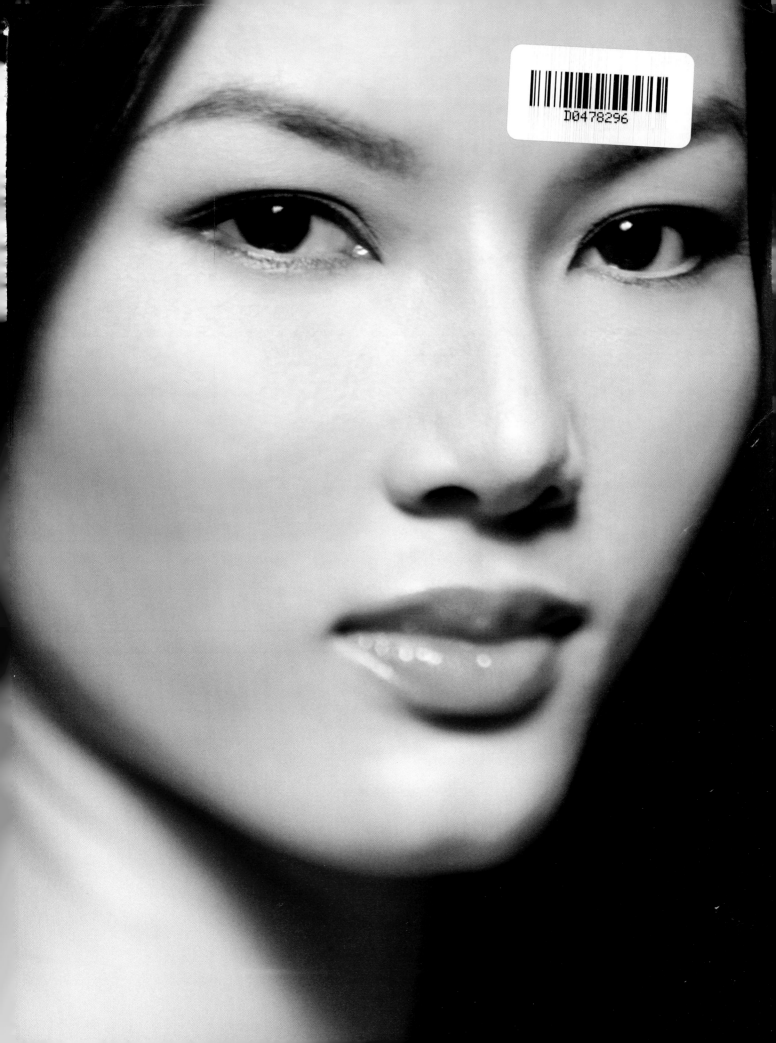

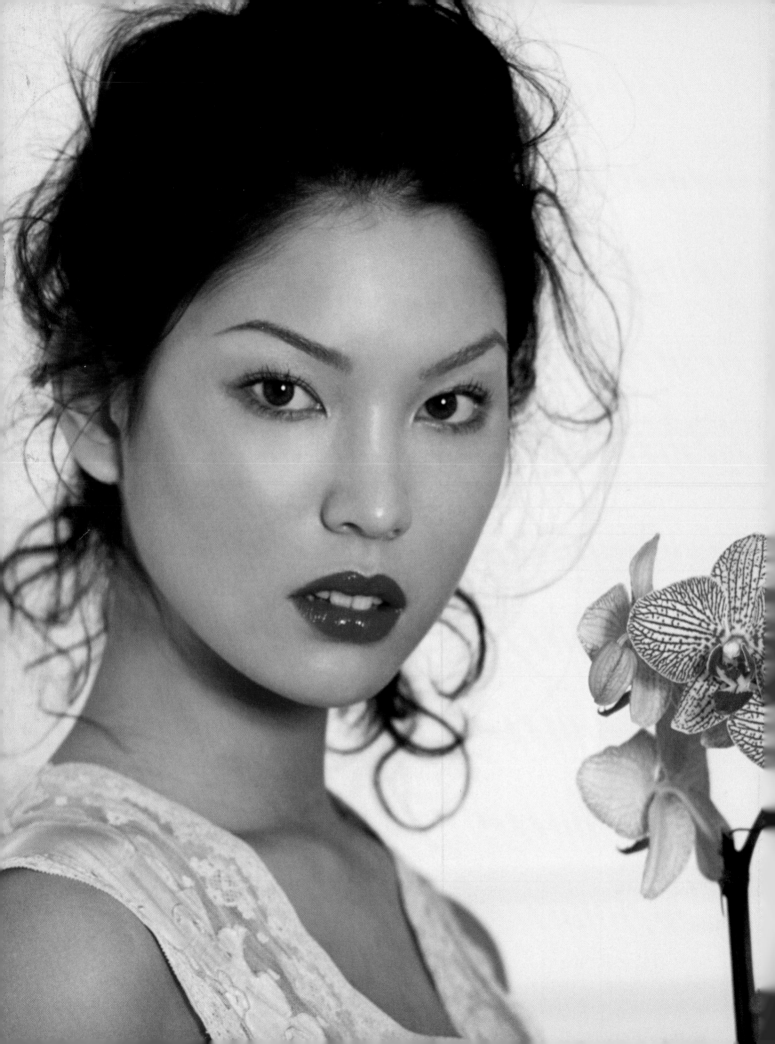

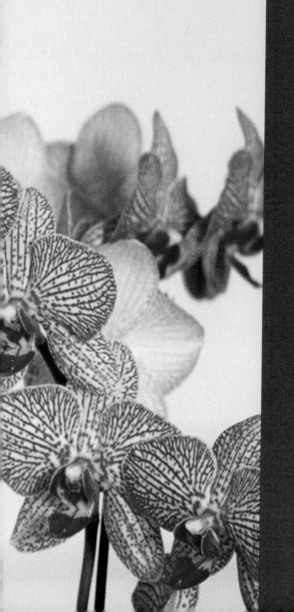

The Essential Beauty and Makeup Guide
for Asian Women

# ASIAN FACES

TAYLOR CHANG-BABAIAN

A PERIGEE BOOK

**A PERIGEE BOOK**
**Published by the Penguin Group**
**Penguin Group (USA) Inc.**
**375 Hudson Street, New York, New York 10014, USA**
Penguin Group (Canada), 90 Eglinton Avenue East, Suite
700, Toronto, Ontario M4P 2Y3, Canada (a division of
Pearson Penguin Canada Inc.) • Penguin Books Ltd., 80
Strand, London WC2R 0RL, England • Penguin Group
Ireland, 25 St. Stephen's Green, Dublin 2, Ireland (a divi-
sion of Penguin Books Ltd.) • Penguin Group (Australia),
250 Camberwell Road, Camberwell, Victoria 3124,
Australia (a division of Pearson Australia Group Pty. Ltd.) •
Penguin Books India Pvt. Ltd., 11 Community Centre,
Panchsheel Park, New Delhi—110 017, India • Penguin
Group (NZ), 67 Apollo Drive, Rosedale, North Shore 0745,
Auckland, New Zealand (a division of Pearson New
Zealand Ltd.) • Penguin Books (South Africa) (Pty.) Ltd.,
24 Sturdee Avenue, Rosebank, Johannesburg 2196,
South Africa

Penguin Books Ltd., Registered Offices: 80 Strand,
London WC2R 0RL, England

Cover photo by Albert Sanchez
Cover design by Liz Sheehan
Interior design by Taylor Babaian and Pauline Neuwirth
Interior photo credits are listed on pages 164–165.

First edition: August 2007

Library of Congress Cataloging-in-Publication Data

Chang-Babaian, Taylor.
  Asian faces : the essential beauty and makeup guide for
Asian women / Taylor Chang-Babaian.
    p. cm.
  ISBN 978-0-399-53314-3
1. Beauty, Personal. 2. Women—Health and hygiene—
Asia. 3. Asian American women—Health and hygiene. 4.
Face—Care and hygiene. 5. Cosmetics. I. Title.
  RA778.C376 2007
  646.7'2—dc22
                                          2007006176

PRINTED IN THE UNITED STATES OF AMERICA

10  9  8  7  6  5  4  3  2  1

While the author has made every effort to provide accurate
telephone numbers and Internet addresses at the time of
publication, neither the publisher nor the author assumes
any responsibility for errors, or for changes that occur after
publication. Further, the publisher does not have any control over and does not assume any responsibility for author
or third-party websites or their content.

Neither the publisher nor the author is engaged in rendering
professional advice or services to the individual reader. The
ideas, procedures, and suggestions contained in this book
are not intended as a substitute for consulting with your
physician. All matters regarding your health require medical
supervision. Neither the author nor the publisher shall be
liable or responsible for any loss or damage allegedly aris-
ing from any information or suggestion in this book.

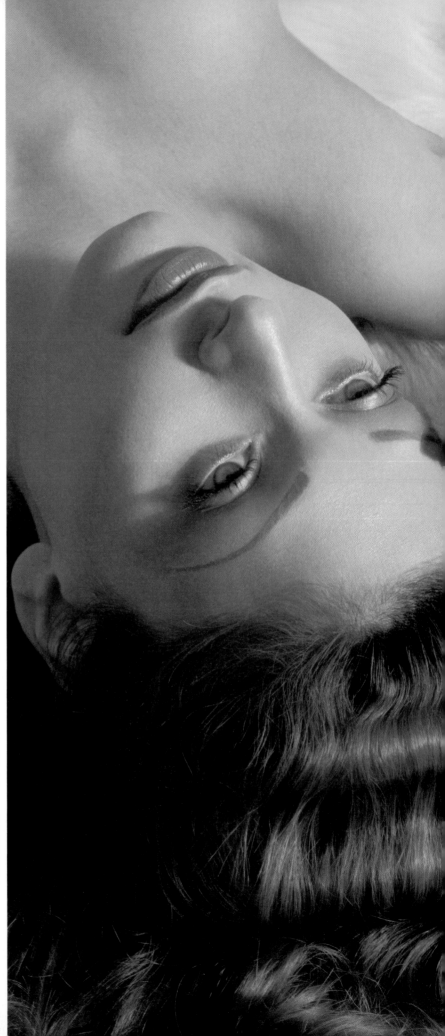

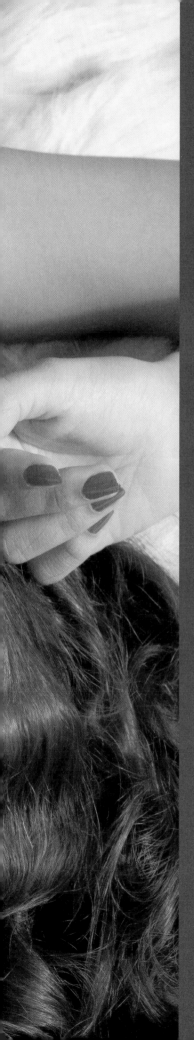

This book is dedicated to all women who, like me in the past, have had a hard time applying makeup. I hope you have as much fun learning new techniques and trying new looks as I do every day.

This book is also dedicated to all of those who believed in me from the beginning and have stayed with me along the way. To my family for always being there, and to my husband, Raffi, and my children, Adina and Christopher, for their incredible support and for always making me laugh.

To everyone at the Cloutier Agency who I can't thank enough for helping get me here. To my friend Hasblady Guzman, who taught me that I can be anything I want to be. To the late Kevyn Aucoin, whose work inspired me, and to all women, whose faces continue to teach me.

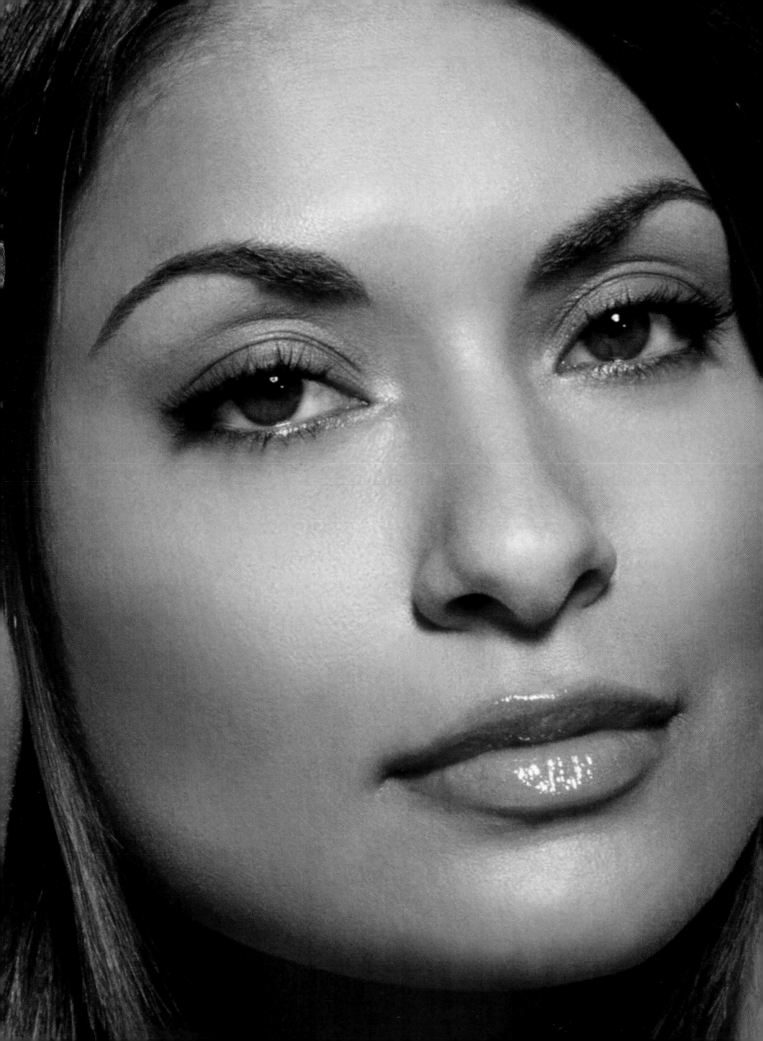

# ASIAN FACES

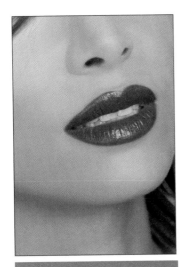

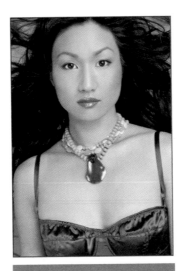

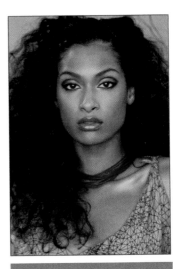

# contents

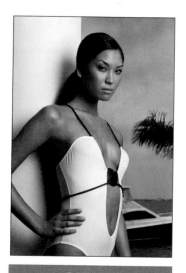

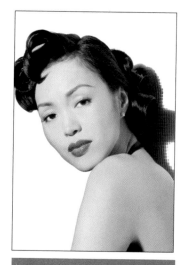

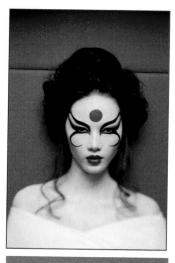

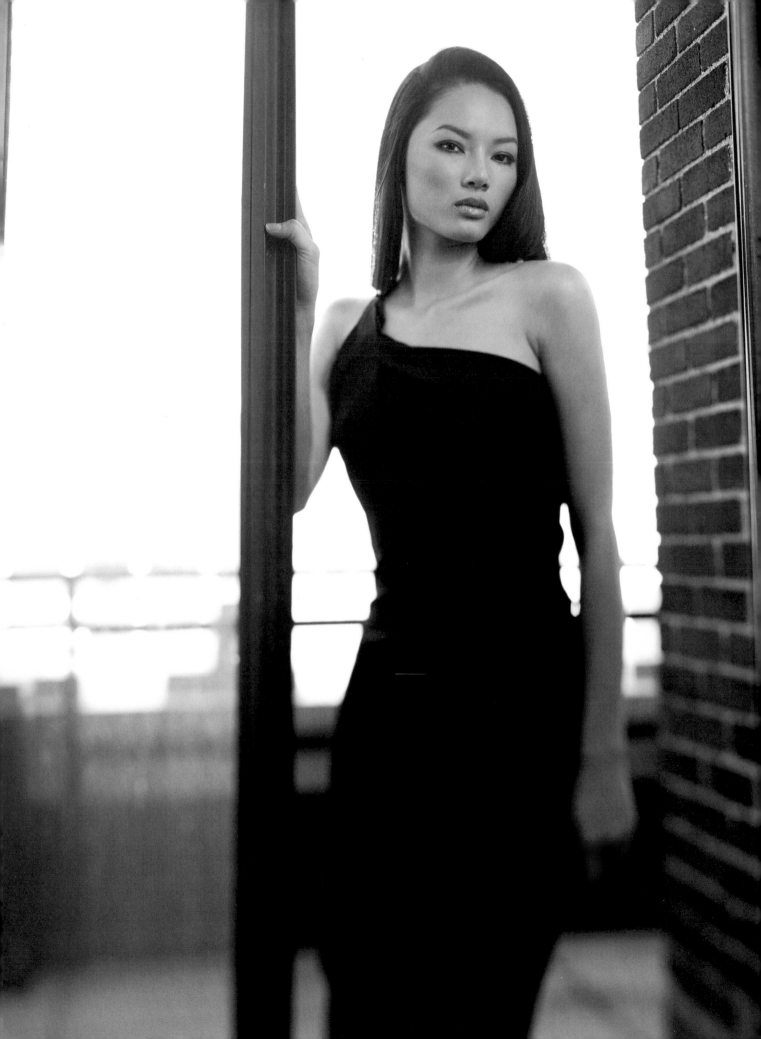

I WROTE THIS book with all Asian women in mind. No two Asian women are alike, and no two Asian faces are alike. The term *Asian* applies to a wide variety of cultures: Chinese, Korean, Indian, Vietnamese...the list goes on and on. And the makeup that works for one woman might not work for her sister. We have so many variations in skin tone, eye shape, and bone structure. That's why it is so important to learn the basics of makeup—why do I apply brown shadow here and shimmer there? How do I make my eyes appear larger or my skin look more even? When you understand what products do and how they work, you will be able to adapt them to your needs and develop the makeup look that is best for you, whether it is a natural look, something for work, or a sexier look for a night on the town. And if you already feel like a makeup pro, you'll learn new tricks, easier application techniques, and fun new looks. I have put everything you will ever need to know about makeup into this book so that you can learn how to be your own makeup artist. Don't get discouraged if it takes some practice—it's just makeup, after all, and you can always wash it off and start again! Take your time, have fun with it, and remember that it is our diversity that makes us beautiful. I am very proud to be Asian, and it has been a lifelong dream of mine to have this opportunity to help all Asian women look and feel their absolute best. Good luck and enjoy!

# YOKO ONO

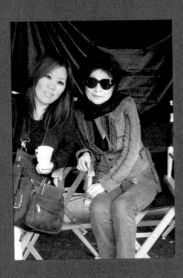

*the author and yoko on set*

WHAT A GREAT BOOK! All Asian women should read this. (I'm just waiting for a pocket-size book to come out so I can carry it around!)

Taylor is so talented and has such an incredible sense of humor. The book is spunky and wise. Only an Asian woman can write this way. Asian women have such a great sense of style that is uniquely their own.

All makeup professionals should read this to know what to do with ASIAN FACES. Because, from my own experience, I know that they often don't!

Finally, all guys should read this to know what fun we Asian women are having. Maybe they would like to join us. Just kidding!

—Yoko Ono
March 20, 2006

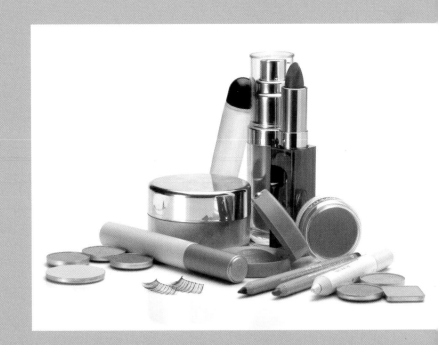

# beauty school

AS A KOREAN child, I had very strict parents, and unlike many girls my age, I wasn't allowed to play with makeup. Then, when I was seven I went through my mother's makeup bag and found a pretty tube of red lipstick and decided to try it on. I was so excited. I felt like such a grown-up, drawing it on just like my mother did. First the upper lip, then the lower lip. Over and over—I must've applied four coats!

I was up on my tippy-toes trying to get myself high enough to see the results in the mirror and admiring my new look when—Aahh!—I heard my mother coming through the front door. I frantically wiped off the cherry red lipstick with tons of toilet paper. (Anyone who's ever tried to remove red lipstick knows you can't get it off in one wipe.) I ran out of the bathroom and pretended to be doing something else. She screamed for me, in the way only a Korean mother can scream. She had seen the red toilet paper in the trash and freaked out because she thought I was bleeding. She made me take off all my clothes and had everyone in the family come into the bathroom to find where I was bleeding. It was humiliating! She finally realized that it was just makeup and of course reprimanded me, but with a sigh of relief.

So, though traumatized by my first lipstick experience, I began to draw. I drew faces. I liked to see what they would look like with eyebrows, without; with eyelashes, without. Fat... Thin... I drew and colored in makeup on my paper models with crayons or shaded them in with pencils or pens. I never thought about why I drew faces until recently. I thought it was just something I liked to do as a child, but now that I'm a makeup artist, it all makes sense.

# makeup

## brows

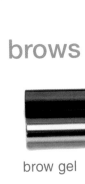

brow gel

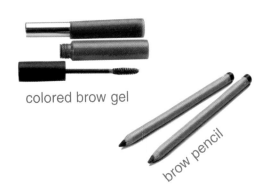

colored brow gel

brow pencil

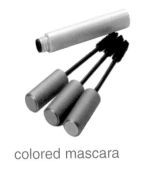

colored mascara

## lips

lip liner

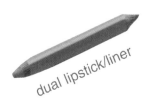

dual lipstick/liner

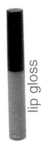

lip gloss

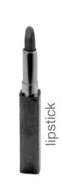

lipstick

## skin

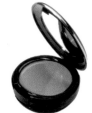

cream foundation

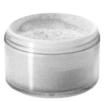

loose powder

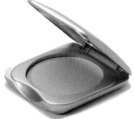

pressed powder

tube

dual

jar

wand

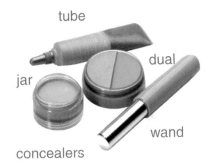

concealers

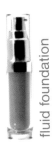

fluid foundation

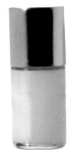

skin illuminator

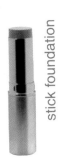

stick foundation

# eyes

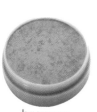
cream eye shadow (stick)

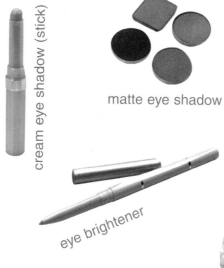
matte eye shadow

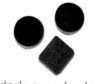
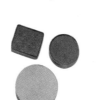
dark eye shadow

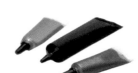
mascara

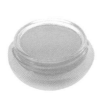
shimmer eye shadow

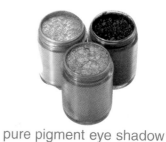
cream eye shadow (tube)

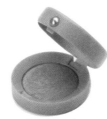
eye brightener

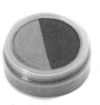
glitter

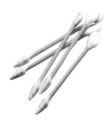
pure pigment eye shadow

# cheeks

bronzer

powder blush

cream blush

dual blush

# tools

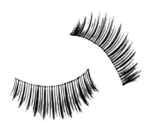
full strip false upper lashes

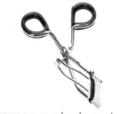
corner eyelash curler

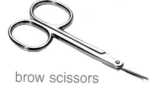
cotton swabs

eyelash comb

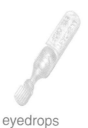
eyedrops

brow scissors

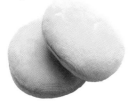

powder puffs

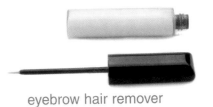

eyelash adhesive

eyebrow hair remover

single hair eyelashes

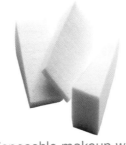

disposable makeup wedges

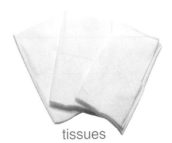

individual eyelashes

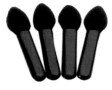

disposable eye shadow applicators

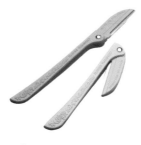

brow razors

tissues

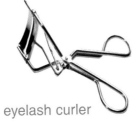

eyelash curler

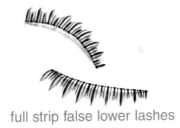

full strip false lower lashes

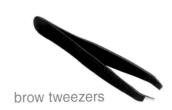

brow tweezers

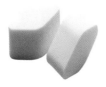

washable makeup wedges

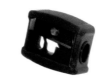

cosmetic pencil sharpener

# brushes

When it comes to your tools, splurge! Good-quality brushes should last you ten years. The right brushes can make all the difference in makeup application. You wouldn't use a screwdriver to hammer in a nail because it wouldn't work. The same idea goes for makeup. You need the proper tools to create the look you want. Make sure that your brushes stay clean so they don't collect bacteria. Use a mild detergent and water (I like to use shampoo) to wash brushes similar to how you would wash your own hair. Rinse thoroughly and lay brushes flat on a towel to dry. You can also use a brush cleaner (sold in beauty supply stores) to disinfect brushes quickly.

## large concealer brush

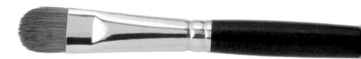

I like to use large concealer brushes for the under-eye area and other large areas that may need concealing. Look for sable or synthetic bristles that are flat and rounded. These brushes are also great for contouring smaller areas like the sides of the nose.

## precision concealer brush

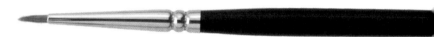

Use precision concealer brushes if you have very small areas that need lots of help. I usually use this brush for sun spots and acne or scarring.

## small concealer brush

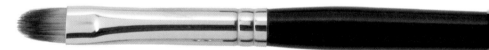

I prefer small concealer brushes for smaller areas that have darkness, usually for small dark circles under the inner corner of eye. These are also great to use with a tiny bit of concealer as an eraser to clean up mistakes around the mouth and under the eyes (see page 28).

## large lip brush

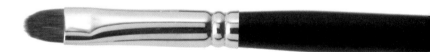

Lip brushes definitely make a difference in creating that perfect lip. I like large ones for larger mouths or if I'm applying lip gloss. Look for synthetic or sable bristles.

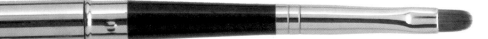

**small lip brush**

The small lip brush is great for smaller mouths, obviously, but I also like to use it to finish off a dark lip look when I want the lines around the lips to be perfect. Look for synthetic or sable bristles.

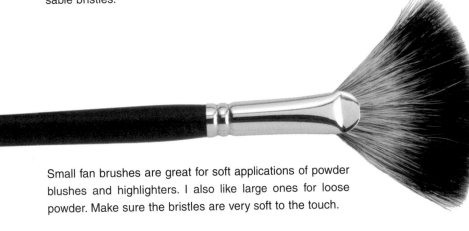

**fan brush**

Small fan brushes are great for soft applications of powder blushes and highlighters. I also like large ones for loose powder. Make sure the bristles are very soft to the touch.

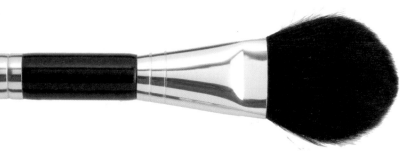

**blush brush**

The blush brush is great for applying color to the apples of the cheeks. I also keep several around for contouring or to use with highlighters. They need to be soft so they don't irritate the cheek area.

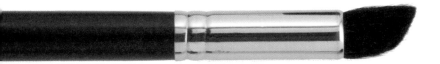

**small powder brush**

I use this brush to powder underneath the eye or wherever else there might be small creases like laugh lines. This brush is great for touch-ups throughout the day.

## large foundation brush

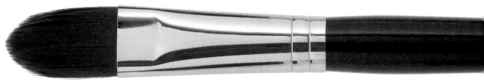

Synthetic is best to absorb less product and go on more smoothly. These brushes are great for contouring and blending foundation. Get a second one to apply cream blush.

## powder brush

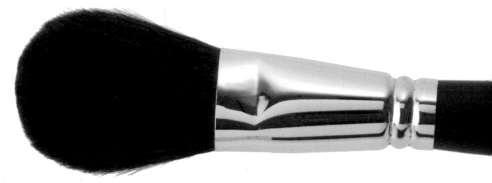

I have probably a dozen powder brushes. You can use them to bronze the face and chest, to softly dust powder to set makeup, or to dust shimmer. The brush you choose should feel heavenly.

## blend brush

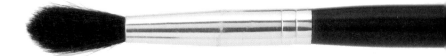

This is great to use to blend eye shadows together. Be careful not to blend the different shadow layers too much, or the color will appear muddy. Especially when you're dealing with the delicate eye area, it's important to buy a really soft brush with long, fine hairs.

## flat shadow sponge brush

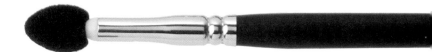

I actually started learning how to do makeup using a sponge brush. It deposits heavy amounts of shadow to the eyelid. They usually have disposable heads, so change them often.

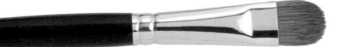

**large shadow brush**

I like to use the flat side of this brush to apply heavier amounts of shadow onto the largest area on the lids (layer 2; see eye shadows). Apply shadow with this brush by gently tapping the brush from side to side on your lid. Always use softer hairs when working with the eye area; most of these brushes are made from goat or sable.

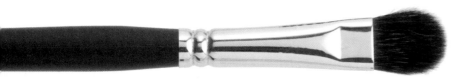

**fluffy shadow brush**

Great for looser, soft applications of shadow, such as applying a soft shimmer.

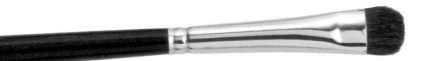

**small fluff shadow brush**

I like to use this brush closer to the base of the lid (layer 3). Look for bristles that are soft and firm, usually made of goat hairs.

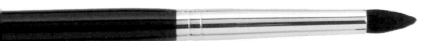

**small shadow contour brush**

Use to smudge thicker amounts of liner to create a smoky effect on the eye. This brush is also great for contouring lids at creases for those with larger double eyelids.

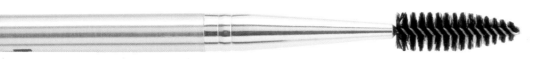

**spool brush**

The spool is a great brush for cleaning up excess mascara. A lot of makeup artists also use this brush for smoothing out fine-to-normal brows or removing excess sculpting gel from eyebrows.

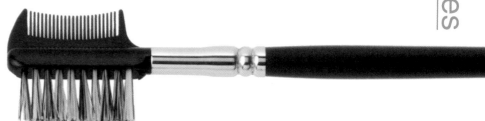

## eyelash comb/ brow brush

Use the lash comb if you've applied too much mascara. The metal ones are finer, but definitely scarier. Metal eyelash combs are incredibly sharp; their teeth look like twelve very fine sewing needles in a row. I've stabbed myself in the finger many times just picking one up. They do separate lashes better, but for safety go for plastic. The bristle brush is great for thicker eyebrows because it gets deeper into the brow layers.

## small angle brow brush

Look for short, semi-stiff bristles to fill in brows with powder. I also like synthetic bristles when working with creams or if I want to create a sharper angle.

## liner smudge brush

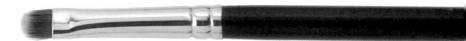

This is a must-have for me. I use it to smudge eyeliner to create an even line. Look for synthetic and short bristles.

## flat liner brush

This brush is great to create lines with eye shadows. It's also great for beginners who don't have the steadiest hands.

## detailed small shadow brush

This is a multipurpose tool. I use it if I want to highlight the inside corners of eyes using shimmer, or as a thick liner brush.

## liner brush

Use this brush for creating lines with gels or cream liners. I prefer the hairs to be semi-stiff for more control and ease.

# cool tips

**forehead** To minimize a large forehead, use contour two shades darker than your natural skin tone, leaving only a small natural area above the bridge of the nose (see page 59).

**temple** Don't forget to apply a small amount of bronzer or blush to your temple in addition to cheeks when adding color to a drab skin tone (see page 55).

**bridge of nose** Apply highlight or concealer here to give the illusion of a narrow nose (see page 59).

**upper lashes** Use waterproof mascara to set lashes longer. Make sure to use a high-quality lash curler—it will make all the difference (see page 48).

**lash line** Use eyeliner along the lash line to give the illusion of fuller lashes. Set with dark shadow for a longer lasting look (see page 51).

**lower lashes** Use waterproof mascara to prevent smudging (see page 48).

**apple of cheek** Place a hint of color here to give life to your face (see page 55).

**cheekbone** Use contour two to three shades darker under the cheekbone to give shape to rounder faces (see page 55).

**jawline** For mature women and rounder faces, contour under the jawline using a color one to two shades darker to give the jaw a more sculpted look (see page 59).

**chin** To minimize a chin use a darker base color; to bring it out use a highlighter in the center of the chin (see page 59).

**collarbone** Add highlighter along the collarbone to accentuate it. To minimize a strong collarbone add bronzer.

**brows** To minimize overplucking, use white eyeliner to cover unwanted hairs first. This allows you to get a preview of what your brows will look like before you actually start tweezing (see page 33).

**brow bone** Apply a highlighter or shadow lighter than your natural skin tone to accentuate the arch in your brows. This gives additional dimension to flat eyelids (see page 42).

**eyelid** Apply shadows by layering the colors from top to bottom with the darkest color closest to the lash line and lightest on the brow bone. This will add depth to flat eyelids (see page 41).

**outer corner of eye** Use eyeliner to create the illusion of a longer and/or larger eye. Using a dark liner on the upper outer corner of the eye gives lift to mature or downturned eyes (see page 51).

**inner corner of eye** Use this as a guide to determine the starting point of your eyebrows (see page 33). Add highlight on the inner corner of the eye to give the illusion of a whiter, open eye (see page 69).

**pupil** Use this as a guide to determine where to begin the arch of your brow (see page 33).

**outer lip line** To make lips appear fuller and to balance out uneven lips use this as your outermost boundary (see page 37).

**inner lip line** To make lips appear smaller or to balance out uneven lips use this as a guide (see page 37).

**upper lip** Most of the time upper lips are much smaller and need balance. Use the outer lip line to guide you (see page 37).

**lower lip** If the lower lip is significantly larger than the upper lip, use the inner lip line to guide you to create a slightly smaller lower lip. This creates a mouth that appears to have balance and looks natural (see page 37).

**center of the lower lip** Place gloss in the center of the lower lip to add fullness and a finished sexy look (see page 15).

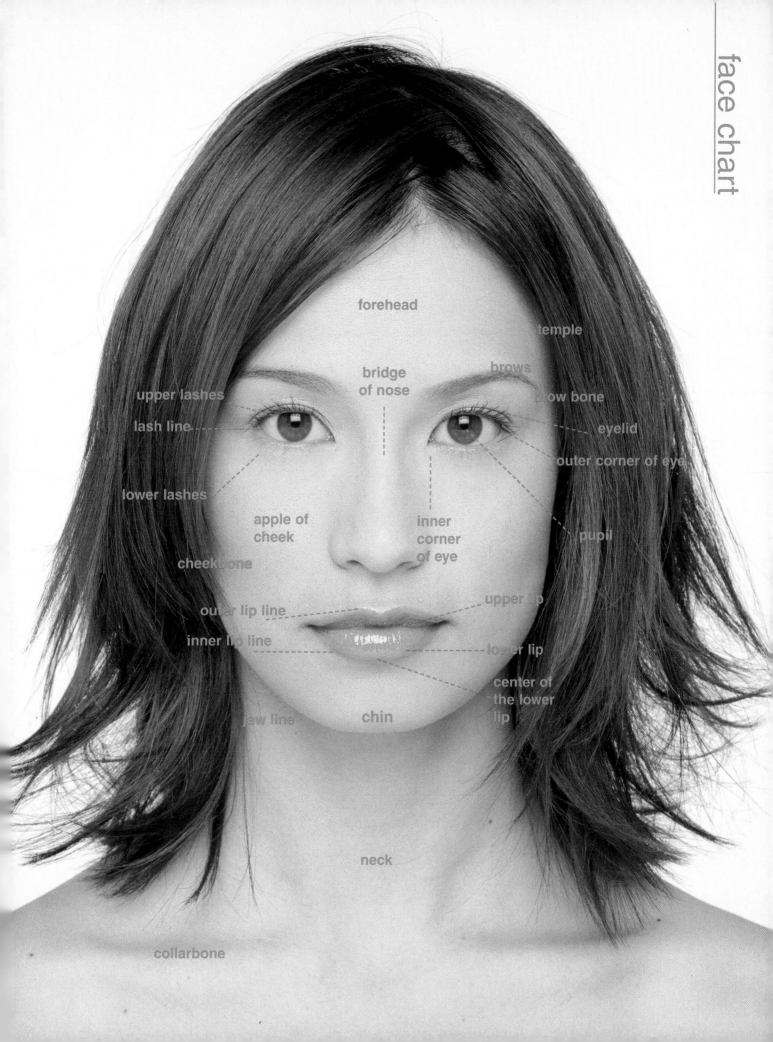

forehead

temple

brows

bridge
of nose

brow bone

upper lashes

eyelid

lash line

outer corner of eye

lower lashes

apple of
cheek

inner
corner
of eye

pupil

cheekbone

upper lip

outer lip line

inner lip line

lower lip

center of
the lower
lip

jaw line

chin

neck

collarbone

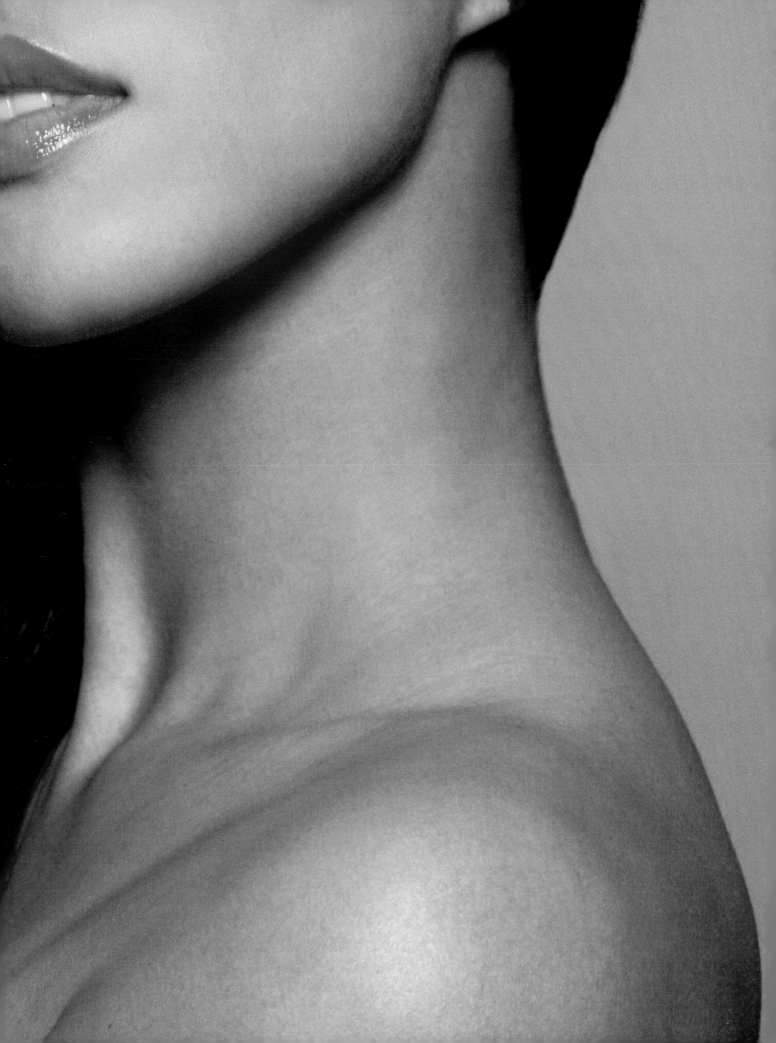

There is more pressure on Asian women to have perfect skin because after all that's what we're known for in the world—beautiful, flawless skin. However, many times that's not the case. Taking care of your skin can be an expensive and tough job, but it is definitely worth it because without great-looking skin, everything else looks messy. Skin changes throughout the year and as we age, so refer to the different skin-type sections whenever necessary.

## See your dermatologist

Although this can be an expensive luxury for many of us, in the long run it can save you money and time. Trying several types of products to self-medicate can be costly and unproductive, especially if you have severe acne, scarring, or hyperpigmentation. There are so many new products today that your dermatologist can fix almost any skin condition.

## Sunscreen

No matter what your age, use sunscreen. It amazes me that so many women today are willing to undergo drastic surgery for wrinkles but don't wear sunscreen. The sun is a major cause of wrinkles, dryness, and hyperpigmentation. I've heard excuses from some women that sunscreens are too heavy for their skin, or that there is no time for any additional product. Sunscreens now come in very light formulas; you'll forget you even have it on. It can also be found in foundations so you don't have to perform an extra step. You really no longer have an excuse not to take care of your skin. Start applying sunscreen with an SPF of at least 15 for the best prevention.

## Hyperpigmentation

Hyperpigmentation is one of the biggest concerns among Asian women. It usually appears beginning in your late twenties to early thirties. This occurs in the skin due to acne scarring, sun damage, a change in hormones as often occurs during pregnancy, even from waxing. Symptoms are noticeable as dark patches on your skin. You can prevent a lot of hyperpigmentation by simply using sunscreen. To fix existing problems, however, there are also many new over-the-counter products that contain ingredients like kojic acid or hydroquinone that are melanin blockers. (Melanin is a pigment that gives skin its color.)

Depending on your situation Retin A or acid peels may be the choice for you. Talk to your dermatologist to find out which works best for your skin.

## Acne

I thought worrying about acne was over once my teenage years were gone, but acne occurs for many reasons: hormones, stress, and environment. Usually acne occurs around the oily T-zone (the area encompassing the forehead, nose, and chin) area in Asian women. Besides it being a nuisance, acne tends to scar more in Asian skin and grow darker, especially if you don't wear sunscreen, causing skin to look even more broken out than it really is. Acne is found in so many different levels of severity that it's recommended you see your dermatologist, as you may not know whether you need to simply wash your face with a new product or you may need stronger medication. If it appears as small bumps you see along your cheek or apples of your cheeks, it could be environmental or from dirty telephones or possibly a dirty brush or sponge. Although it is constantly debated that what you consume does not affect your skin, I would have to strongly disagree. Your skin is an organ and I've found that minimizing caffeine intake, drinking more water, and doing cardiovascular exercise has made all the difference in helping to clean out my pores and keeping my skin looking youthful and clear. It definitely can't hurt. No matter what the case, be gentle to your skin so that you minimize the potential of scarring, and do your research. Keep skin clean and dirt-free by washing at least twice a day. Give new products recommended to you a chance; many times you'll have initial breakouts because of the underlying clogged pores before you'll notice skin starting to clear. And remember to always use a light oil-free sunscreen.

# how to wash your face

I remember watching my mother as a young girl going through her morning and evening ritual. One by one she'd put on her foam washes and expensive creams. I know everyone thinks they know how to wash their face, but you would be surprised. I met one girl whose concept of proper cleansing was wiping her face with petroleum jelly and cotton pads. This is definitely not the appropriate way to wash your face. Although the products for each individual may change, the routines are usually the same.

If your body's skin is as thick as one hundred sheets of paper, then your face is the thickness of ten sheets of paper and your eye area is like one sheet of paper—so treat them accordingly. If you're seeing a dermatologist, make sure to ask about your cleansing routine as they may require these steps to be in a different order. Remove eye and lip makeup first, and then wash your face. Don't forget to wash your hands before touching your face.

## 1. Cleanse

Test the water for temperature; it should be warm, but not hot! Then close your eyes and gently splash warm water onto your face to loosen dirt and makeup. When your face is nice and damp use your fingers to rub in cleanser in a circular motion. Don't forget your jawline and harder to reach areas like the sides of your nose.

Use warm water to rinse cleanser off, and repeat if necessary. I like to do a final rinse with cool water (not cold, as this could pop capillaries, which are the little pink veins you may see on your face).

Then gently pat your face with a towel—don't rub!

## 2. Treatments

This is usually an evening step. Skip this step in the morning unless directed differently by your dermatologist.

### Exfoliate

Apply exfoliant (usually a form of acid derived from fruit enzymes and used to remove dead skin cells) onto a cotton pad and wipe over the face, avoiding the eye area.

### Treatment

Do treatments once or twice a week instead of exfoliating. This includes hydrating and clay masks.

## 3. Tone

Sometimes exfoliants are called toners. However, toners actually have a different function. Toner is a product not readily used in America, but it should be. It's a watery substance that you gently slap onto the face. It contains various hydrating substances and does a few things—the light slapping brings blood flow to the skin's surface and the product hydrates the skin and creates a deep glow from within.

To apply toner, create a shallow bowl with the fingers on one hand, and pour a dime-sized amount of toner into the bowl. Then clap your hands together a couple of times and gently slap them onto your face, avoiding your eye area. Repeat if necessary.

## 4. Moisturize

Seal in the glow and use a moisturizer with SPF in the morning and a treatment moisturizer in the evening. Moisturizer can be light for normal to combination skin or thicker for dry or mature skin.

Apply to the skin in circular motions and don't forget to apply to the neck as well.

## normal

Congratulations, you have normal skin! Normal skin is something most of us women strive for. You are a rare and fortunate type, but that doesn't get you off the hook for skin care. You still have to think about damage prevention because skin does change. Just because you have normal skin now does not mean that it won't change throughout the year, becoming drier in the winter and oilier in the summer, so refer to the other skin-type sections when necessary.

### Products to look for

#### Cleanser

Use mild cleansers that don't strip your skin of its natural oils. This is a great preventative to dry skin in the future.

#### Exfoliant

This product may be unnecessary for you because you're probably fifteen years old. (Just kidding—I'm a little jealous!) However if you are very young, your skin is probably turning over its cells right on time and doesn't need any help from exfoliants. As you get older, use a mild exfoliant to remove dead skin cells.

#### Treatment

Look for a clay mask to use once a week to remove impurities and blackheads.

#### Moisturizer

Use a light moisturizer that contains sunscreen of at least SPF 15.

#### Foundation

Use a sheer foundation to even out skin tone if necessary. I prefer oil-free ones that are silicone- or water-based. A little bit of sheer foundation adds an illuminating skin effect that's great for evening looks. Note that even if you have perfect skin you still need to use a little foundation and powder on eyelids to create a base for eye shadow. This makes the shadow last much longer.

#### Concealers

You probably don't need concealer either, but for that annual pimple, I like to use cake concealer in very small quantities. It covers completely but because you don't need to use much of it, others can't even tell you have it on.

#### Powders

You probably don't need this as your skin is practically flawless but sometimes it's nice to have a little fun with powders. Use sheer powders that contain little to no color.

## oily

Although oily skin may seem like a problem now, you might actually be thankful for it later. I've noticed women who have oily skin tend to have fewer wrinkles and continue to look younger longer. However, here are a few tricks to control oil in the meantime.

### Products to look for

#### Cleanser

Use gel cleansers to give oily areas a squeaky-clean feeling.

#### Exfoliant

Use an exfoliant containing alphahydroxy or salicylic acid, concentrating on the T-zone (forehead, nose, and chin) area. If you have acne or need an exfoliant that contains a stronger substance like prescription glycolic acid, talk to your dermatologist.

#### Treatment

Oily skin can attract dirt more that other skin types so take extra care to keep it clean. Look for a clay mask to use once or twice a week to remove impurities and blackheads.

### Moisturizer

Use oil-free moisturizers that contain sunscreen—doubling up moisturizer and separate sunscreen can make your skin feel greasy.

### Creams

Use mattifying creams on the T-zone before applying foundation to control oil.

### Foundation

Use an oil-free foundation to even out skin tone if necessary. I personally prefer to use stick or cake foundation on oily areas and to blend it so it's a very thin coat. Because it requires little product to provide strong pigment, stick or cake foundation can feel lighter on the skin. It also holds on to oily areas better. You can also try using a heavier pigmented powder foundation if you are truly very oily and don't like foundation.

### Concealers

Use cream or stick concealers as they'll hold on to oily areas better than liquid concealers.

### Powders

Use powders containing silica or cornstarch to absorb excess oil and set makeup.

### Blotting paper

Use blotting paper on the T-zone to pick up excess oil throughout the day.

## combination

Combination skin is very common among Asian women. You're likely to have patches of dry, oily, and normal skin. Often this will include an oily T-zone (the area encompassing the forehead, nose, and chin).

### Products to look for

#### Cleanser

Use gel cleansers to give oily areas a squeaky-clean feeling.

#### Exfoliant

Use an exfoliant containing alphahydroxy or salicylic acid, concentrating on the T-zone area. If you have acne or need an exfoliant that contains a stronger substance like glycolic acid, talk to your dermatologist.

#### Treatment

Look for a clay mask to use once a week to remove impurities and blackheads.

### Moisturizer

Use oil-free moisturizers that contain sunscreen—doubling up moisturizer and separate sunscreen can make your skin feel greasy.

### Creams

Use mattifying creams on the T-zone before applying foundation to control oil.

### Foundation

Use a sheer foundation to even out skin tone. I prefer oil-free ones that are silicone-based.

### Concealers

Use cream or stick concealers as they'll hold on to oily areas better than liquid concealers.

### Powders

Use finely milled sheer powders to set makeup. For extra-oily T-zone areas, use powders that contain silica.

### Blotting paper

Use blotting paper on the T-zone to pick up excess oil throughout the day.

# sensitive

You generally know if you have sensitive skin. Many products cause you to break out in rashes easily or maybe your face turns red even at the lightest touch. Sensitive skin can be very difficult to work with because it can also be prone to acne and dry patches. Look for exfoliants derived from lactic acid, but talk to your dermatologist first.

## Products to look for

### Cleanser

Look for mild cleansers that are specifically for sensitive skin or whose descriptions contain key words like "gentle." Many companies today have products aimed directly at women with sensitive skin.

### Moisturizer

Look for fragrance-free, colorant-free, and allergy-tested products. Many products will say that they are made for sensitive skin, but it's still wise to look for these specific guarantees.

### Foundation

Use a light foundation to even out skin tone if necessary. If you are very sensitive to foundation, you may opt for a heavier pigmented powder for coverage instead.

### Powders

Loose powders may be better for your sensitive skin as they don't contain the binding ingredients or oils that pressed powders usually do and can be found in lighter textures.

### Brushes

You may be allergic to certain animal hairs. If so or if you are unsure, use synthetic brushes that are very soft. If the bristles feel at all rough, the brush is not soft enough. There are many synthetic brushes on the market today that are even softer than animal hair. To avoid irritation, wash brushes often using a shampoo that you are not sensitive to and rinse them thoroughly, laying them flat to dry. Change sponges and puffs often; as with all skin types you can contaminate your skin by using dirty puffs. Many puffs and sponges can be washed and reused as well. Look at the package instructions or ask your favorite makeup artist.

> **Cool Tip**
> Look for cosmetic products that contain minimal ingredients. See your dermatologist about harsher products like treatments and exfoliants. You may be allergic to specific ingredients.

> **Cool Tip**
> Test products on a small area of the skin (like the back of the jawline) before committing to a product.

# dry

I think there is a common misconception that all Asians have oily skin. Many Asian women have dry skin, whether due to aging, changes in weather, or genetics. It's especially important to take care of dry skin as neglecting it can give you the appearance of heavier lines, especially on your forehead, cheeks, and eye area.

## Products to look for

### Cleanser

Try a mild cream cleanser that doesn't strip the skin of its natural oils.

### Exfoliant

It's important to use exfoliant on dry skin as it helps to renew the skin's surface by sloughing off dead skin cells. Choose an exfoliant that contains alphahydroxy or salicylic acid. It'll give you the look of renewed skin. If you have acne or need a stronger exfoliant, talk to your dermatologist.

### Treatment

Use hydrating masks to give intense moisture to the skin once or twice a week.

### Creams

Use creams that contain key hydrating ingredients like hylauranic acid to multiply the moisture in your skin. For extremely dry, chapped skin, use barrier creams that seal in moisture. There are many barrier creams on the market today; they are ultra-heavy creams that contain ingredients like shea butter and are great for chapped wintertime skin. Look for products that are described as being for "chapped" or "cracked" skin.

### Moisturizer

Apply moisturizer quickly while skin is still slightly damp after washing the face to help the skin absorb the moisturizer. Make sure to use moisturizer before foundation, but wait to let the heavier moisturizer settle, as applying foundation too quickly after moisturizer can cause separation in some liquid foundations.

### Foundation

Use liquid foundations to even out skin tone. Tinted moisturizers are also a great way to speed up the morning routine. Avoid moisturizers whose descriptions contain words like "mattifying." Look for key words like "hydrating." I recommend foundations with a little shimmer to add life to dull skin.

### Concealers

Use cream or liquid concealers under the eye area because thicker concealers can look cakey on thin, dry skin.

### Powders

Use sheer, light powders to set liquid foundations.

# take it off

It may seem odd that I'm writing a whole section on makeup remover, but it's only because I find it incredibly important, especially since many of us need to use waterproof makeup products on our eyes. It's important to find good, gentle removers to protect delicate areas and prevent infections.

## Eyes

The area around the eyes is the most delicate area on the face. The eyes are often the focus of a makeup look. When dealing with layers of eye shadow, eyeliner, waterproof mascara, and false eyelashes, it's important to take all this off carefully, making a gentle and effective eye-makeup remover vital. Look for oil-free removers that say specifically they are made to remove waterproof makeup. Apply remover to a cotton pad and remove eye makeup using a gentle touch. I use cotton swabs for the hard to reach areas like under the eyes. You can also use pads that are pre-soaked in remover and remove excess oil with cotton pads. I find tissues a little too rough for that area. I like to remove all eye makeup first, and then continue with my routine.

## Lips

I usually remove lipstick and lip gloss using a clean tissue. If there is still any leftover stain, I apply petroleum-based lip balm and let it sit for a few moments, then wipe it off with a tissue. There are also specific lipstick-remover lotions that you can use. For really tough dark-hued lipstick stains, try using a little eye-makeup remover.

## Makeup Wipes

I like makeup wipes, not baby wipes, for a temporary solution. They're great as a last resort to remove excess dirt if you are not near water or only want to remove a specific portion of your makeup. For example, you're at the office and need to remove caked foundation and redo it without ruining your eye makeup. However, I personally prefer cleanser and water whenever possible.

## Exfoliants and Astringents

Use exfoliants to remove all excess dirt that your cleanser may not have picked up. Avoid the eye area. After cleansing your face, use a cotton pad to apply astringents to your face and neck. You'll notice it helps to tighten pores by removing dirt and oil. I like astringents that contain a little witch hazel or alphahydroxy or salicylic acids.

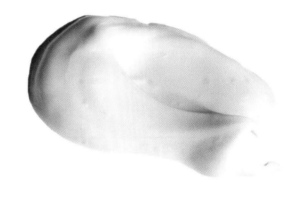

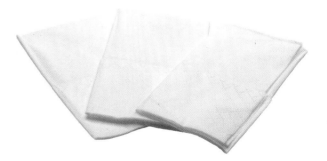

# foundation

Foundation can be the hardest cosmetic product to find, especially for Asian women. Our skin comes in so many different colors, from the palest olive tones to very dark with olive undertones or very dark with slightly red undertones (our skin is neither red nor olive; undertone means there is a hint of the color as the underlying base). In the past, foundations were predominately found to have a pink base. Thankfully cosmetic companies wised up and realized skin does not only come in light pink, and now most companies have a wide variety of foundations with yellow and olive tones available for Asian women. With proper foundation it's easy to see your most beautiful features. Your beautiful eyes are not competing with a pimple or uneven skin tone. When your skin looks flawless, suddenly your features are more obvious. You look awake, refreshed, and youthful.

**Cool Tip**
The best light to see if you have on the right foundation is natural daylight.

## Choosing the Right Color

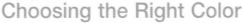

You've heard all the crazy places to test foundation—the wrist is very popular—but the best place to test your color is on your jawline. This way your foundation will blend with your neck. Choose a few different foundations that you think are a close match and apply them vertically on your jawline so that you can see at least an inch of each color. Look in the mirror, holding it about a foot away from your face so that you can see the overall picture. The foundation you choose should seem almost invisible because it blends so well into your skin. I have never met an Asian woman with pink skin, unless it was because of a skin irritation, so please stay away from pink foundation. Look for foundations that have a yellow undertone for light to dark skin. Look for yellow or a slight olive undertone for very pale skin, and for very dark skin, match jaw line and neck then use a lighter color for the center of the face (forehead, nose, under the eyes, above cheeks). I like to match the color just directly under the eyes. (For very dark skin, see contouring section.)

## How to Apply Foundation

Before applying foundation, always prep skin with moisturizer, otherwise the foundation will look blotchy and

**I've never liked heavy face makeup. Although it is necessary for film and heavy lighting, most people don't need it for everyday life. During the day, I like to wear as little as possible—usually just a little concealer. However, for an evening look, I go all out. I use a sheer base, concealer, and powder to give myself flawless skin so that I can create a dramatic look. Doing this draws attention to the focal point you create, which for me are usually the eyes and lips.**

cracked. If your skin is oily, use astringent to clean off dirt and oil, then moisturize and follow with foundation.

No matter what tool you decide to use to apply the foundation, it's all applied the same way: DOWN. The fine hairs on your face grow downward, so you want to apply foundation in the same direction to make them less visible. I like to start from the forehead and work my way down. Apply foundation to your chosen tool and swipe in a downward motion from the center to the sides of your forehead. Work your way down the nose and along the sides of the nose, adding more foundation in small amounts as necessary. For the eye area, start from the inner corner of the eyes and move to the outer corner, blending gently. (Applying foundation to the eyelids helps in the even application of eye shadows and makes them stay on longer.) Don't forget the temples. Continue applying foundation downward from the cheeks and under the nose and chin. Blend into the neck, so there is no line of demarcation, conceal any still-visible blemishes, set the whole look with powder, and *voilà!* perfect skin.

**Cool Tip**
Allow moisturizer to settle into skin for a few moments before applying foundation to ensure better coverage.

## Primer

There are many types of primer on the market—some are more for a better foundation application, others are meant to fill in pores; some do both, and some do nothing. If you choose the wrong primer it can leave foundation looking blotchy. To avoid bad results use the same brand of primer as your foundation. If you want to try it out, ask about return policies or take your foundation with you to try the combination at the counter.

## Tinted moisturizer

This product provides the sheerest coverage—just a hint of color added to moisturizer. Most do come in yellow-based tones and they are so sheer that they blend with most skin tones. This is great for someone who doesn't need much coverage and has very little to no acne, or for mature skin that needs just a bit of color. It's also great for those in a huge hurry. Most tinted moisturizers contain moisturizer, sunscreen, and some color, so you get three steps covered in one product.

## Sheer foundation

The lightest substance in the foundation family, this is great if you have fairly good skin tone and just need a little help evening out your overall color. I prefer silicone bases as they mix well with most moisturizers and work well with dry to oily skin.

## Liquid foundation

This type of foundation is generally found in a bottle. It comes in a variety of textures from very sheer to heavy, full coverage. I prefer liquid foundation for mature or dry skin as well as skin that needs only minimal coverage but has some redness.

## Cake foundation

This foundation is found in compact or stick form and gives the most amount of coverage, as it has very dense pigment. I prefer cake foundation for very dark skin as well as oily skin. Because of its consistency and dense pigment, you can use very little and it is less likely to slide or melt off of oily skin.

## Cream foundation

This usually comes in pots or tubes and has a thicker consistency but still provides a wide variety of coverage, from light to heavy. However most of the time it contains more pigment than liquid foundation so you need to use less of it to get the same coverage.

**Cool Tip**
When creating a smoky eye, clean up stray eye shadow using cotton swabs and apply your foundation afterward.

## Foundation Tools

Yes, on top of worrying about color and texture, you need to make sure that your foundation tool is right for you. Different tools give a different effect to foundation.

### Wedge sponge

This is great if you have a hard time with blending. Sponges release less product, making it easier to blend. Apply foundation directly onto the sponge and spread over the face as outlined in the "How to Apply Foundation" section. You can also use sponges to blend out foundation if you've applied too much using the other tools. On the downside, sponges absorb product so you are likely to go through your foundation twice as fast. Buy disposable sponges for the most sanitary usage. If you have more expensive reusable sponges, wash them regularly, paying attention to their washing instructions. (They usually need to be washed in warm water with a mild soap.)

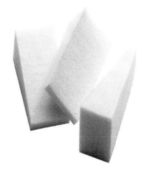

### Your fingers

The cheapest method will often give you the heaviest application. The heat of your fingers warms up the foundation and helps it blend more easily into the skin. Make sure your hands are clean, using soap and water before working with any product. Apply foundation onto your fingers and, using small quantities at a time, spread foundation onto your face. Of course, it can be a bit of a mess. If you've just gotten a manicure you may want to opt for another method.

### Foundation brush

I feel like Picasso when I use this brush. It is usually made of synthetic fibers and because it absorbs little to no product it affords you a lot of control over the application. Choose a brush that thins out at the tip. I prefer synthetic fibers made of high-quality taklon. Wash this brush regularly, following manufacturers instructions. (They usually need to be washed in warm water with shampoo.)

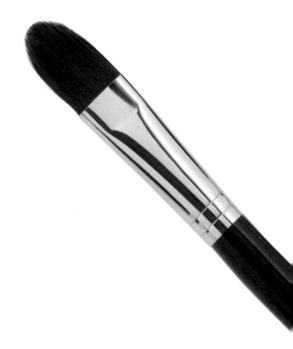

## Tricks of the Trade

Now that you've learned the basics of foundation application, here are some insider tips.

### Building on Foundation

This is simply applying another coat of foundation. Just as you would apply a second coat of paint when painting a house, you put on a second coat of foundation on your face. However, this isn't paint and you're not a house, so when you apply a second coat, you only want to add it where necessary (i.e., if you have red cheeks, apply the second coat there). After applying your first layer of foundation, wait a moment before applying the second layer so your skin has time to absorb the first coat. When applying the second coat, do not apply downward as you did with the first coat, as you're likely to rub off the first coat. Instead gently pat a small amount of foundation on to the necessary areas using quick, short taps, working slightly around the targeted area to ensure a nice blend.

### Using Two Different Shades

When purchasing your foundation I generally recommend buying the next shade up or down as well (depending on what time of year it is). You're never just one color throughout the year unless you're truly very good about staying out of the sun (using sunscreen, a hat, shades, and an umbrella regularly), which most of us aren't. You will more than likely get paler during the harsh winter months when the sun is not so strong and darker in the summer when sun is harsher and you're more likely to do outdoor activities. You can use the lighter foundation during the winter, the darker for summer, and mix the two for the months in between. Once you become more comfortable with applying foundation, you can use the different shades to add contour to your face. If you're using the lighter shade of foundation, use the darker under the cheekbones to define them. If you're using your darker shade use the lighter foundation along the middle of your nose as a highlighter. (This makes your nose look narrower without looking like you obviously thinned out your nose.)

> **Cool Tip**
> If you forget which foundation to use for contouring, just remember that dark shades make features recede, while light colors bring features out.

### Severe Acne

If you have severe acne or oily skin and everything slides off, try dusting on a full-coverage powder instead of foundation, then use a small brush to conceal excess redness.

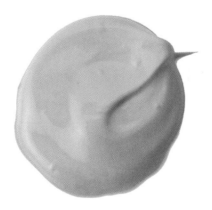

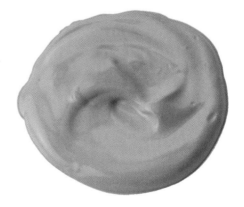

# concealers

I think all women are on a constant search for that perfect concealer. What they don't realize is that even if they find one, their needs will change over time. With your skin texture constantly changing due to environment or mood, your concealer will need to change, too.

## Make the Look Flawless

I was in Asia a while ago reading one of the current beauty magazines, when I felt sick to my stomach. They had written up a brand of concealer as the best concealer of the year. The same concealer I had written up many times, but not for Asian women. Make sure when you read "Best Beauty Product" awards they're referring to products that work for Asian women, not just the masses.

I almost always use two different types of concealers: one for the thin skin underneath the eyes and another concealer for the face to cover up acne, sunspots, or any other imperfections. Concealer can be tricky because if it's too light, you look like you have a halo around the imperfection. If it's too dark, you've created more darkness and drawn more attention to the area.

If the imperfection is pink or red, use a concealer with a yellow undertone; if it's black (for example, a mole), use one with a pink undertone; if it's blue (for example, under eye circles), use one with orange undertones. Concealers should be applied with your fingers or a small concealer brush (I prefer synthetic short brushes made of high-quality taklon) for precise coverage. When purchasing concealers, it's best if you have your foundation on so that you can match the concealer to the foundation.

For under the eyes, I often lighten the dark areas using a thinner, more fluid concealer. This minimizes wrinkles and darkness without looking cakey. If you're young or have dark skin, you can use a stick or cake concealer.

For imperfections around the nose, chin, and forehead, I prefer concealers that are thicker, usually in stick form, or in a pot or palette. This prevents the concealer from running. The shade should be about half a shade lighter than the skin.

### Cake concealer

This stuff is intense. Cake concealer is very dense in texture and opaque in coverage. I prefer cake for oily skin and to cover imperfections in the skin, like scarring or acne.

### Pen concealer

These concealers are very light in texture but can cover light to medium dark circles. They're usually best for dry skin or fine lines under the eye or if other concealers are

## Cool Tip

Apply concealer after foundation and before powder. That way you use the smallest amount of concealer necessary and the concealer won't move around because you've already applied the foundation.

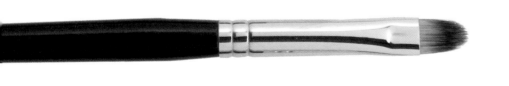
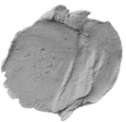

too cakey for your skin. However, I have never seen pen concealers for darker skin, which is fine because I prefer creams for darker skin anyway.

## Stick concealer

This medium-to-heavy coverage concealer has similar texture to a cake concealer but is usually less dense. I usually don't even use a powder after applying this concealer, and if I do it has to be very sheer. This is my choice for warm weather, or if you have a problem with concealers staying put.

## Treatment concealer

This is similar in consistency to a pen concealer and usually comes in a pen or wand (the same ones lip gloss comes in). The concealer contains fruit or salicylic acids and antibacterial medication for the treatment of acne. For best effect, use a small brush or cotton swab to apply powder to the blemish after applying the concealer. Since the product is very thin, there's greater risk of it moving around on the skin so apply it gently and only use it on areas with acne, but not around the eye area. See your dermatologist to treat severe acne.

## Cream concealer

I like this creamy butterlike texture better for the under-eye area as it contains more moisture and is great for concealing dark circles. It provides medium to heavy coverage and comes in a tube or pot.

## Tattoo cover concealer

This heavily pigmented concealer is definitely an insider secret and is also used for perfectly covering moles, freckles, blackheads, and scarring. These are the heaviest of concealers and are specifically designed to cover tattoos. I once covered a girl's tattoo and she had forgotten what her legs looked like without it. I've actually had two occasions where models have shown up on set with a black eye and this covered it perfectly, so the client never knew.

**Cool Tip**
For the best coverage on the under-eye area apply concealer directly to the dark region and gently blend it using your finger.

# powder

The first powder I used came in a brown compact and was a light pink. It was a horrible match for my skin—you could see it from a block away! Today, you can set makeup with powders that are almost invisible. Powders come in a wide variety of colors and textures, from very sheer types to heavy foundation and powder combos.

## Setting Foundation

Setting foundation is basically applying powder on top of liquid foundation so that it sets into skin. This is important because you don't want the foundation to move after you've spent time applying it to perfection, and due to your body heat or in warm weather it is sure to run. The trick is setting it so it doesn't look heavy or obvious. This is where a lot of women go wrong. The foundation starts off looking great and suddenly you've aged twenty years because you've applied too much powder. (With no foundation, powder alone doesn't have the same aging effect.) If you have great-looking skin a little concealer under the eyes and a dusting of powder is probably all you need.

## Choosing a Powder

Different powders and tools will give you a different effect depending on your skin type. For oily skin, look for powders that contain silica or cornstarch to absorb excess oil. With dark skin, I always use two different colors to set foundation because darker women usually have several different skin tones. The forehead tends to be a lot darker than the apples of the cheeks, and the forehead may have a red undertone where the apples may have an olive undertone. Very dark women do have to accommodate their skin tones and use a lighter powder for the center of the face and a darker color for the outside of the face like around the hairline, temples, cheekbones, and jawline.

### Pressed powder

Pressed powder is definitely the best type of powder to keep with you during the day. Most pressed powders contain oils and binding agents to hold the powder in place. If you apply powder outside of your home, it's the least likely kind to get everywhere, especially on your clothes. Thank goodness for makeup technology!

### Loose powder

Loose powder creates a youthful finish and is a great choice for sensitive skin because it doesn't contain a lot of the extras like oils that are necessary in pressed powders to keep the powder in a pressed form. This is my ideal choice—the sheerer the better—using just enough to set foundation. Loose powders come in a variety of colors and are easier to match to skin because they can be applied so lightly that you see the skin coming through. They do also come in heavier forms for more coverage if necessary.

### Wet/Dry powder

This is usually found in compact form. It's basically a heavily pigmented, very dense powder. Great for Asian women who want a matte finish with coverage but hate the feeling of foundation. Apply it dry for medium coverage; to apply it wet, dampen a clean wedge sponge with water, squeeze away excess, and apply to skin for heavy coverage. After it dries it's set.

### Translucent powder

Available in loose and pressed form, a true translucent powder has no color or bulk to it at all and creates the sheerest setting for foundation. I like it for light to medium skin tones, but for darker Asian women it can look a little ashy if it has any sort of white pigment to it. I prefer ones that are finely milled and preferably in loose form with a tiny bit of yellow undertone for Asian women to create the most natural look.

### Under-eye powder

Using a finer powder (one with a very soft texture) for under the eyes is essential if the skin under your eyes has fine lines or is dry. More and more companies have developed specific under-eye powders.

### Wet powder

This is fun new technology. This powder looks like normal powder but feels cold and wet to the touch and is a great skin refresher when applied. However, it does mix oddly with some foundations that contain oil or silica. I recommend using it with a water-based foundation. I've also seen it in bronzer form. Wet powders have a sheer finish—great for hot summer days or pregnant women who need to feel cooler constantly.

## Powder Puff

Puffs will deposit too much product if you let them. To get a lighter application of powder, pick up powder with the puff and rub off the excess powder on your other hand. This way you control the amount of powder you use. To apply it to your face, press the puff gently onto the skin in a rocking motion (picture a boat in the ocean rocking in waves). Puffs are great for traveling, touching up at work, or during a night out on the town.

## Brush

Using a brush is my favorite way to apply powder, as it gives the most controlled application and deposits a small amount of powder. This way you still look natural and not cakey. Choose a large powder brush and make sure it's high quality and really soft. Your best options are brushes with hairs made of taklon (a high-end synthetic fiber), goat, squirrel, or sable. Avoid rough brushes; not only will their bristles irritate skin, they will not deposit powder evenly. Pick up powder using your brush, shake off any excess by lightly tapping the handle with your finger close to the bristles, and apply powder in a downward motion going along the growth of the hair of your face. Make sure to keep brushes clean (see page 9).

## Touching up Oily Skin

I wanted to touch on this point because I've noticed that when Asian women get oily during the day they go straight to the powder and apply it directly on top of the oil, usually on and around the nose, forehead, and chin. This is a mistake, especially when using colored powders because if they are applied to an oily surface the powder will darken and the oily areas will appear to be darker. Instead, use something to blot off excess oil, such as tissue or blotting papers (I prefer ones that don't have powders on them already) before reapplying powder. If you also need to reapply foundation or concealer, apply a small amount of concealer to cover any imperfections (concealers that are in a stick or cake form will hold on to oily skin better than a liquid concealer), then finish with powder (look for powders that contain silica or cornstarch, as they'll absorb access oil).

**Cool Tip**
For sheer powder applications use a large powder brush. For heavier applications use a powder puff.

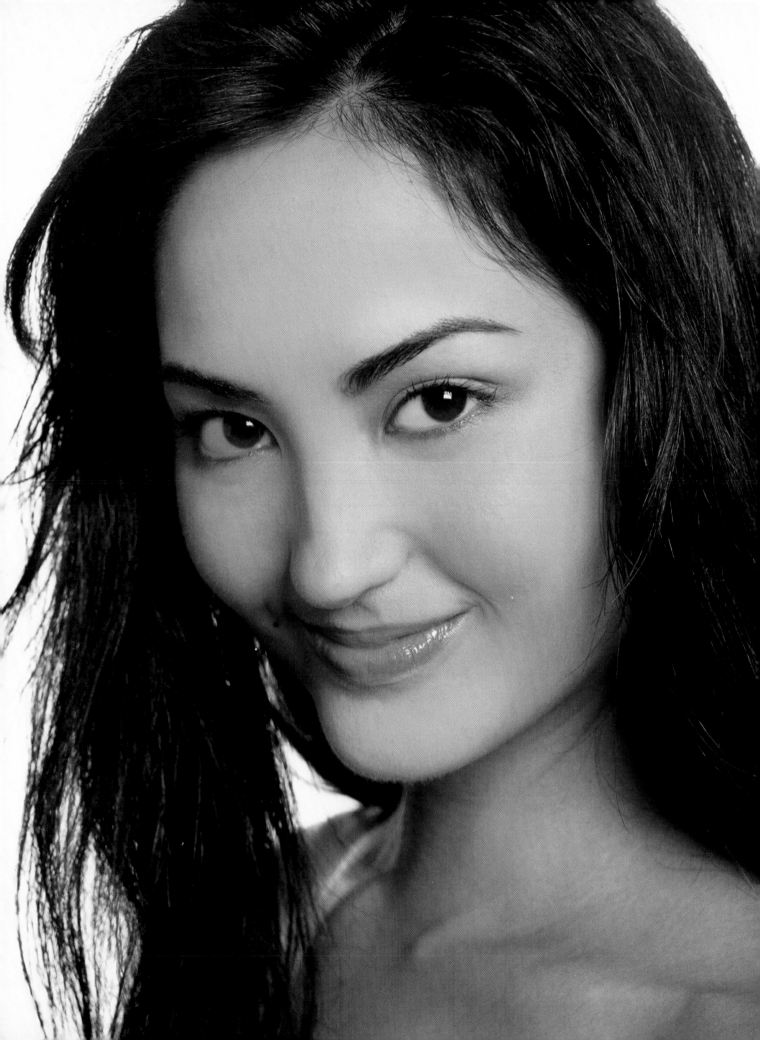

# brows

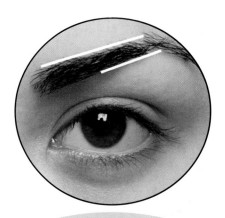

When I was little and drew faces for fun, I always drew them without eyebrows. I didn't see the purpose in them. As I got older, though, I realized how important eyebrows really are. Eyebrows add expressiveness and symmetry to the face and eyes.

Asian eyebrows can grow like crazy—up, down, and everywhere. So here's a few tips to help define unruly brows.

**a**
Brows should begin here. Place a pencil (eraser-side up) vertically along the side of your nose and slightly outside the corner of the inner eye.

**b**
The arch begins above the outside of the pupil.

**c**
To determine where the brow should end, place a pencil (eraser-side up) diagonally from the nose to the end of your eye. The brow should end at the point the pencil hits.

**d**
For wide-set eyes, start brows closer to the bridge of the nose.

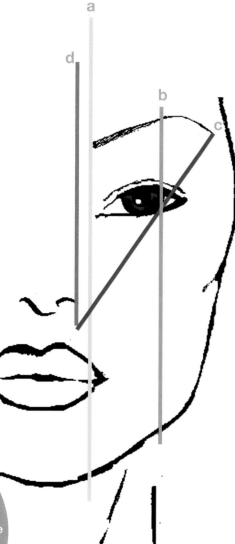

### Cool Tip
Asian brows tend to be sparse at the ends of the brows so make sure to pay attention there. If some hairs are questionable to tweeze, move hairs around to see what removing them would do, then tweeze.

**Use** white liner to determine tweezing area. (Cover stray hairs with liner to see how brow will look once they are tweezed.)

**Tweeze** above and below the brow.

**Brush** brows up and cut excess length, going against the growth of the hair.

**Many times** the ends of Asian women's brows grow down. When cutting the underside of the brow, brush hairs down and carefully cut into a perfect arch. (You may have to cut the ends first before tweezing some of the unwanted hairs under the arch and end of brows.)

**Look** for scissors with short blades to avoid accidental overcutting.

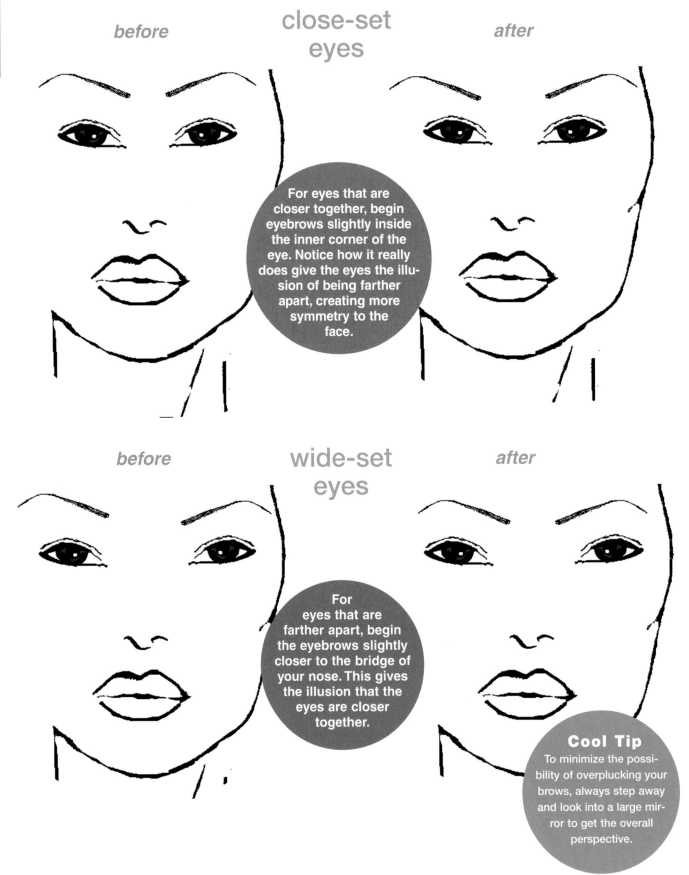

*before*

## close-set eyes

*after*

For eyes that are closer together, begin eyebrows slightly inside the inner corner of the eye. Notice how it really does give the eyes the illusion of being farther apart, creating more symmetry to the face.

*before*

## wide-set eyes

*after*

For eyes that are farther apart, begin the eyebrows slightly closer to the bridge of your nose. This gives the illusion that the eyes are closer together.

**Cool Tip**
To minimize the possibility of overplucking your brows, always step away and look into a large mirror to get the overall perspective.

The look of your brows can change according to your makeup style. For example, when I want to create smoky eyes and light lips I usually make my brows appear defined but definitely soft, whereas when I want dark lips and light eyes I prefer a slightly darker brow. This is based on preference, so you should make your own choices depending on what type of look you prefer.

### Tweezers

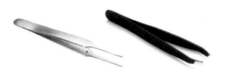

You get what you pay for when it comes to tweezers, so make an investment and buy a professional brand. Tweezers come in slanted, flat, and pointed shapes. The pointed style is best for those really hard-to-get hairs, but be careful—they're sharp! I like the slanted style best as you can get rid of the hairs fast. Stick with the flat heads to apply false eyelashes.

### Scissors

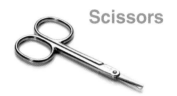

Asian brows have a tendency to be more difficult to control and to grow downward at the ends. You will need scissors to cut the hairs correctly and create the proper shape. I like small, straight scissors, preferably stainless steel. Look for types made specifically for brows with short blades to avoid overcutting.

### Clear brow gel

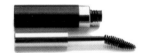

Use brow gel to set your finished look, especially if you have not yet trained your eyebrows to stay in place. Use the gel sparingly and don't touch your brows after they're set. Messing with them too much can make the gel flake off.

### Brow cream

This is a fairly new product. I use cream when I want a defined, strong brow. It is especially great for filling in very sparse areas. If you want a more natural look be careful to use the cream sparingly, as it packs a powerful punch with just a little product. It's best to apply it with an angled brow brush.

### Brow brush

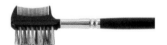

This is an essential tool that I use to train brows to stay up or to brush brow hairs up or down before cutting them. This brush usually comes in the shape of a toothbrush or a spiral. I prefer the spiral shape for thinner brows and for more detailing of brows and the toothbrush shape to brush up full brows.

### Brow pencil

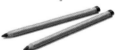

Brow pencils generally last longer because they usually contain waxy ingredients. They are great for creating sharp lines at the ends of brows.

### Brow powder

This is the best product to create softer-looking brows. I like to use powder at the beginning of the brow and a pencil for the end of the brow to create a soft, defined brow. Powder is best applied with an angled brow brush. You can also use eye shadows as brow powder.

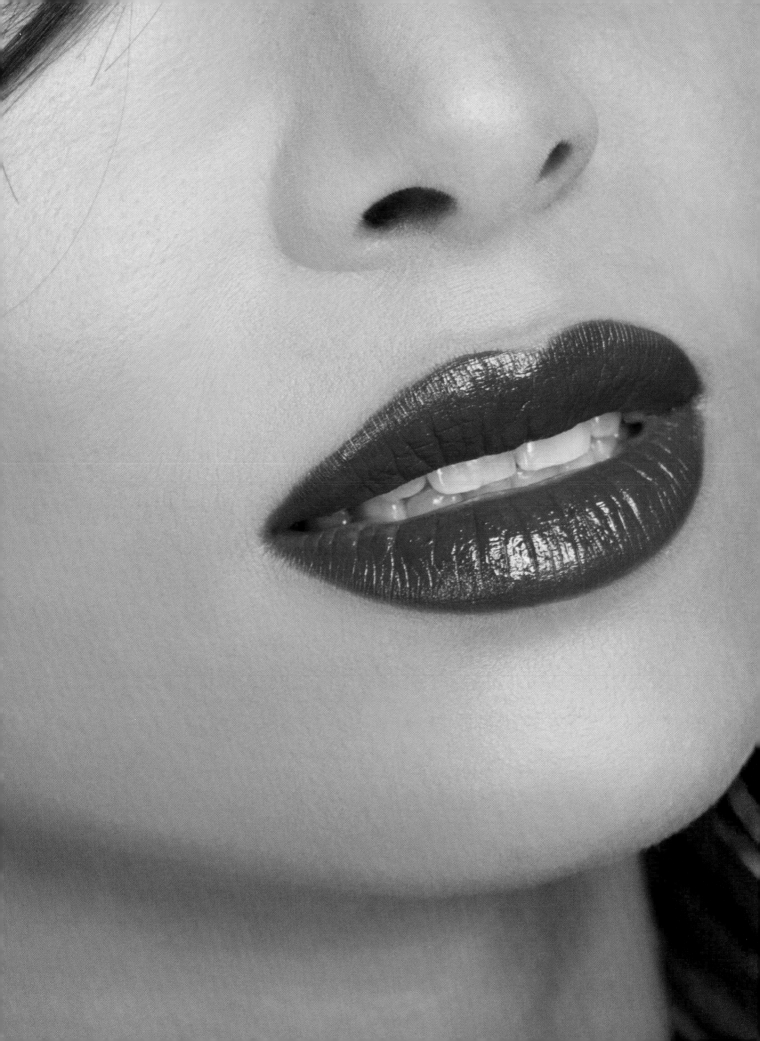

When changing the natural lip line to create the illusion of a smaller or larger mouth, it's important to keep it looking subtle and natural. I recommend a lip liner that is one or two shades darker than your natural lip line. Even for red shades I often use a neutral lip liner and go over it with my lip color choice. When making lips appear smaller make sure to go over the natural lip line with a little concealer to hide the lip's natural shape. For lighter colored lips, where lip colors can look bright, look for colors that are warmer (more brown). Darker lips tend to have more blue to them, so look for cooler colors (more pink).

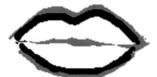

**To create the
illusion of a
smaller mouth**

**draw the line
on the inside of
the lip line**

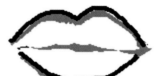

**To create the
illusion of a
larger upper lip**

**draw the line
slightly above the
top lip line**

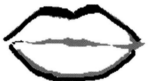

**To create the
illusion of a
larger lower lip**

**draw the line
slightly below the
bottom lip line**

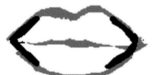

**To create the
illusion of a
shorter mouth**

**draw the line
inside the corners of
the lip line**

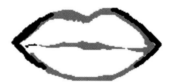

**To create the
illusion of a
wider mouth**

**draw the line
slightly outside the
corners of the lip line**

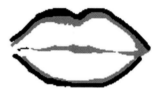

**To create the
illusion of a
larger mouth**

**draw the line
slightly outside
the lip line**

To balance out Emily's lips I drew the lip liner line slightly above the top lip line to create the illusion of a larger upper lip.

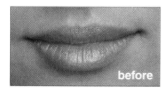

before

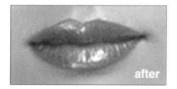

after

**Cool Tip**
Use warm shades of lip liners to add richness to lipsticks and lip glosses. This allows you to use that pink that may have been too bright on its own.

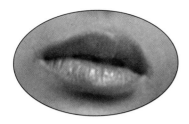

## Natural lip

The natural look is great paired with a smoky eye and looks effortless. Use nude lip liner and sheer lipstick to create this look.

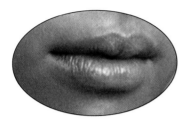

## Nude lip

This is a great high-fashion look, but it should be paired with a fairly dark eye so that you don't look washed out. Apply foundation or concealer onto bare lips and follow with a nude lipstick or gloss.

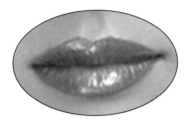

## Warm opaque lip

This lip look is great for a warm, bronzed style and works well with either light or dark eye makeup. Use a warm lip liner to darken shades and follow with lipsticks or glosses in gold, copper, and other warm shades.

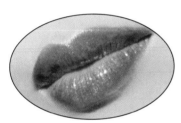

## Sheer glossy lip

This look is sexy but sweet and is great with a natural to medium eye makeup when using darker lip colors, and it's great with almost any eye when using neutral colors. You can also use almost any lip color and add a lot of clear gloss to it to create a sheer gloss. Use lip liners to add definition to the mouth if necessary.

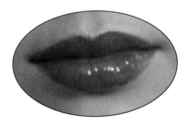

## Dark opaque glossy lip

This has to be paired with a neutral eye and executed very well, especially when bright lip colors are involved. This is definitely a technique for the advanced makeup junkie. Look for berries and reds, pinks and purples. Think of the '80s.

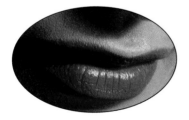

## Matte lip

I love this for period looks (as shown here for a 1930s-style shoot). It's great to use in cool and warm reds and brick hues.

**Cool Tip**
To clean up lipstick mistakes, add concealer to a small brush and use it as an eraser.

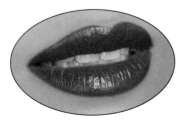

## Creamy lip

This lip look has just a slight sheen but is opaque and gives off a lot of color. These lipsticks are great for a classic, sophisticated look. Great in neutral pinks, mauves, berries, reds, and bronzes.

You can find lipsticks, creams, and glosses nowadays in pretty much every different shade, texture, and packaging imaginable. Choosing one depends on your style and preference. I love them in neutrals, apricots, warm pinks, and deep reds.

## Lip balm

Lip balm is a true must. Use it before any lip color application to create a smoother surface. I prefer one with SPF 15.

## Matte lipsticks

Matte lipsticks are usually more opaque and dry. They are great for both strong and minimalist looks. Mattes are used often in period styles, usually in redder tones. If I'm looking to create a strong red lip I usually choose one with a matte texture. When coupled with a clean, natural eye the result is a strong look that didn't require too much makeup.

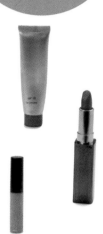

## Cream lipsticks

Cream lipsticks are great for those who always have dry lips. They add moisture without also adding too much shine.

## Sheer lipsticks

Sheer lipsticks are truly the choice for natural lip looks. Usually very creamy in texture, they are more transparent than cream lipsticks. You're less likely to have buyer's remorse with sheer lipsticks because your natural lip color will show through and look great.

**On mature skin, lip color has a greater tendency to bleed, so use lip gloss only on the center of the lower lip and rub lips together once or twice gently.**

## Lip gloss

Lip gloss is truly my favorite because it creates an instant sexy vibe. Whenever I feel a look doesn't have enough kick, I add lip gloss and the problem is immediately solved.

## Dual lip pencil

This is a great product for women on the go or someone who doesn't have a lot of makeup bag space. One end of the pencil is a liner and the other end is a creamy lipstick. The ready-made combination is a plus for those who don't know which liner goes with which lipstick color. They come in so many colors now that you're bound to find one that's right for you. I love technology!

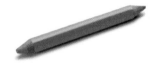

## Lip liner

This is a multipurpose makeup tool. You can use it with lip balm to create a matte lip color and also to create the illusion of fuller or symmetrical lips. I generally prefer neutral lip liner in a slightly darker shade than your natural lip line even if it is used with darker lip colors. You can use a wider range of lipstick and lip gloss colors when you use a lip liner that is at least one or two shades darker than your natural lip color. However, I do often use a warm brown tone to warm up bright lip colors to make them more wearable. Lip liner is also a must to minimize bleeding.

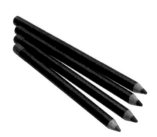

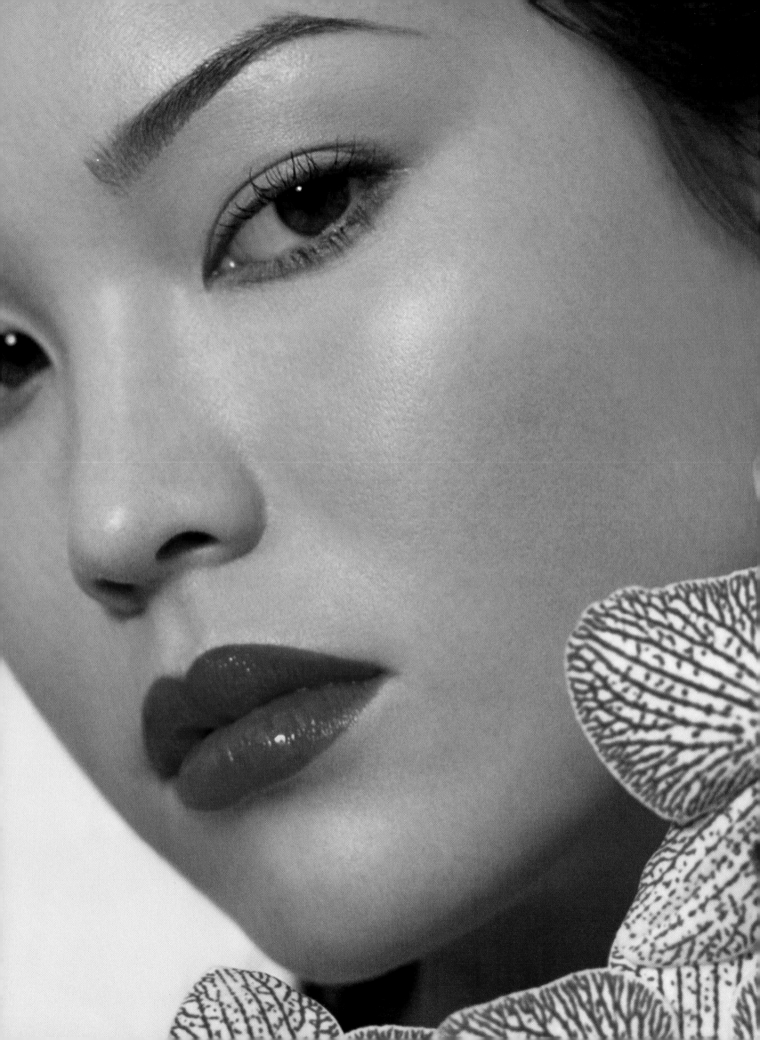

The shape of most Asian eyelids are flatter than other women's eyes. That's not a bad thing. You can change your look so much because you have a lot of lid space to work with. You just have to know what to do and how to do it.

To create depth, I like to work with eye shadow in layers, with the darkest color closest to the lash line, neutral tones in the middle, and highlight colors at the top to accentuate the brow bone.

You can apply only one color of shadow or layer up to four different shadows. Going beyond that is unnecessary.

Eyeliner is a key item for Asian eyes because we can use eyeliner to create the illusion of different eye shapes and to create focal points and depth. It's also useful to make lashes appear fuller.

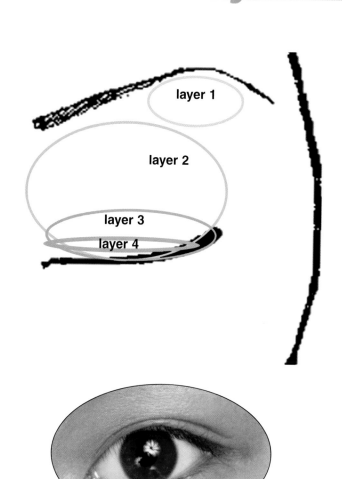

## Eye Shadow

Notice on Emily that the different color eye shadows give her eyes a completely different look. For the day look the copper eye shadow is used in layer 2. This makes her eyes look bright, even the pupil looks lighter. For the evening the green eye shadow is blended into layer 3, with a hint of black liner inside her lower eyelid and smudged under the eyes to give her a smoldery look. Two totally different looks but both are beautiful.

For under the eyes, continue to work in layers. For multiple layers work upside down. Layer 4 closest to the lash line, then layer 3, then 2. Of course this needs to be done in very thin layers, given the limited space. Then I like to use layer 1 in the inner corner of the eyes only (optional).

### Cool Tip
When using several different shadows work around layer 2. This is the shade you'll see the most of.

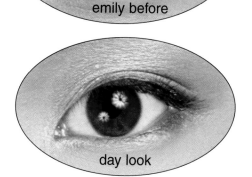

emily before

day look

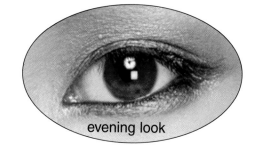

evening look

# eye shadows

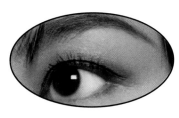

## Bright

Use brighter shadows in layer 2 or layer 3—not both. Soften the brightness with a brown shade in layer 3 or with a smudged eyeliner. For a more natural look, keep shadow on top lid and closer to the lash line.

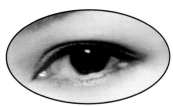

## Natural

I think we all want to look natural in our everyday lives. In order to do so but still look defined, you need to use neutral shadows, with not too much shimmer or color. Stick with taupes, mauves, and browns.

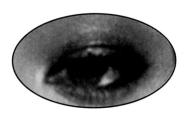

## Smoky

This is actually a very easy look to create. It's important that you just work with layers (see page 42–43) with the darkest layer at the base of the lash line. Pair this eye makeup with a neutral lip to make a fashion statement. Use different shades of brown eye shadow for a more natural daytime look.

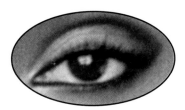

## Contoured

I do not like contouring eyes that don't already have a double eyelid unless it's for a specific look, usually costume. It doesn't make your eyes look any bigger the way layering does. Here the contouring of the lid creates a dramatic effect because I used dark cream shadow. You can do a natural look with more neutral tones.

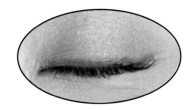

## Clean but strong

This is just one color of eye shadow on the base of the lid (layer 2). Notice how the look is very simple but still has drama.

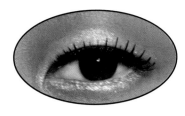

## White halo

This is a strong version, but this look is widely used throughout this book in softer applications. I love using shimmery colors around the whole eye in gold and bronze tones. It makes the eye color pop. You definitely need to team it up with a defined, thin line of eyeliner on the top lid to add depth and definition to the eye.

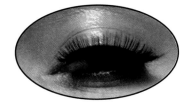

## Glossy

You have to have a certain personality to pull off this look, because it's definitely funky. If you want to try a glossy lid for evening wear, I recommend lighter colors—even clear looks great. Make sure the gloss is designed for use on the eye area.

The eye shadows of today have greatly improved from our mother's eye shadows. Some eye shadows now even contain antioxidants and light reflectors. And the color choices are endless! Here's a guide to help you make the right choice for the look you want.

## Cream shadow

Cream shadow comes in sheer to opaque colors from natural tones to dark purple and is easy to apply with your fingers as your body heat helps to soften the shadow for a smoother application. It's great to use alone for a natural eye look. Apply cream shadows on bare lids for the best results. If you have oily lids, stick with cream-to-powder shadow.

## Loose shadow

Loose shadow usually comes in a shimmery form and can be a little messy at first but it's the best for controlling the amount of color you want. They don't contain any binding agents so they tend to be very light in texture. Use a small brush to apply highlighter loose shadow in white, opal, or gold to the inner corner of your eyes. Use a large brush and shake off excess for a sheer application of pinks, golds, mauves, or pale purples to create an angelic look.

## Pressed shadow

Pressed shadows are my favorite type of shadow because they're the best for layering colors, not to mention they come in colors and textures from sheer shimmers to opaque matte black. You can even find some that contain green tea extracts and antioxidants. I prefer finely milled shadows that are silky and soft in texture.

## Stick shadow

Stick shadows are basically cream shadows in stick form but some do have a tendency to be a little denser in texture because of the shape they have to hold. I find them to last longer than regular pot shadows (cream shadows usually found in small glass jars). Stick shadows are also great because they can be used as shadow or eyeliner and can be applied very quickly.

## Pure pigments

Pure pigments come in loose shadow form and are pure color. They contain very few ingredients other than pigment so they deliver more intense color. They're great for dramatic looks. I like to use them for runway styles or for a fun evening out. Remember to use a small amount and build up from there because a little goes a long way. I prefer dark intense colors like brick, greens, and purples whenever I want a dramatic look.

## Gel shadow

Gel shadows are the newest technology of all the shadows. Like stick shadows, gels can be used as a liner or shadow, but gels usually come in more intense colors than creams and are great for highly dramatic looks when used as a shadow. You must work fast though, as once this stuff sets it doesn't move. My favorite is to use dark brown and black as an eyeliner.

## Cream to powder

Cream-to-powder shadows are longer lasting than cream shadows. They start as an easy-to-blend cream and set to a powder. These shadows are great for those who have oily lids but want a cream shadow. Apply a powder shadow on top for even longer staying power. Great in soft colors like golds and pinks.

**Cool Tip**
When doing a smoky eye, clean up fallen shadow using cotton swabs and eye makeup remover, and apply your foundation after.

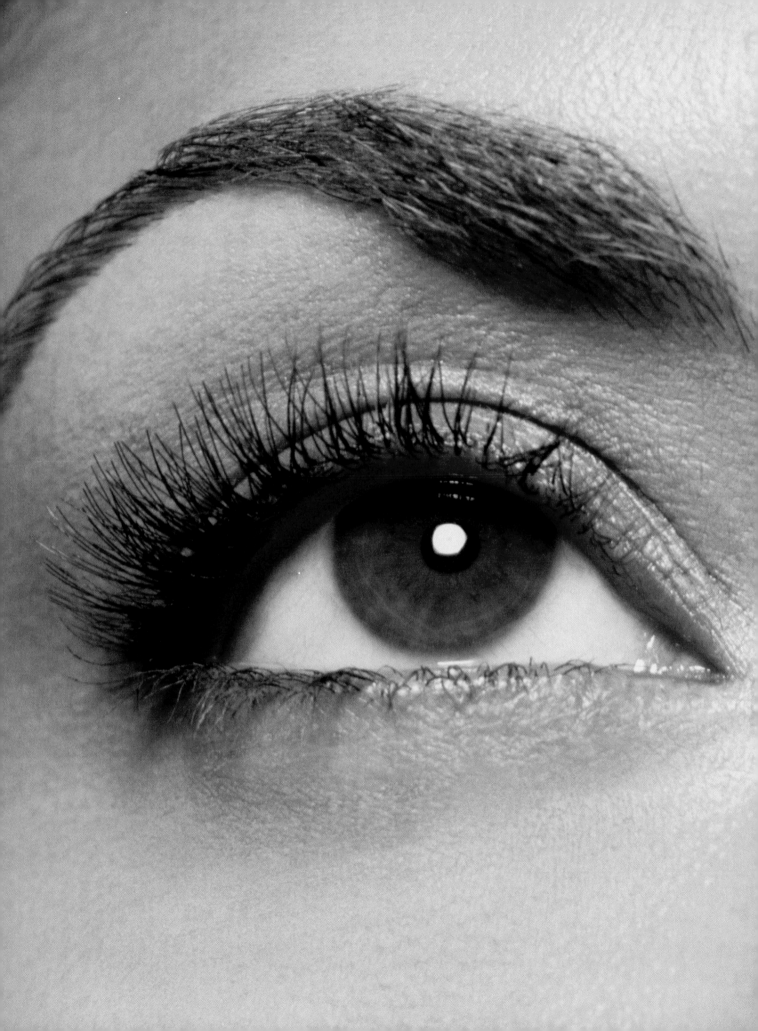

# *false* eyelashes

I get asked a lot about false eyelashes, mostly because they seem nearly impossible to apply to Asian eyes and they look so great on us. They really make a difference in the way our eyes look. The most important thing to remember when applying eyelashes on Asian eyes is that the base of the lashes must be applied as close to your lash line as possible. To do so, look down when applying lashes. This makes it look more natural. For those of you who don't have a double lid, like me, lashes should also be applied away from the inner corners of our eyes (when eyes are open they will still appear to start at the beginning of the lash line, they just won't poke). I also prefer to apply eyelashes last, after the rest of the eye makeup is done. Applying eyeliner or shadow with the lashes already in place moves the lashes and loosens them.

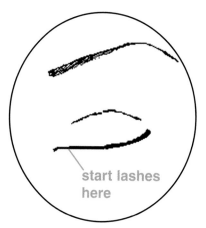

**Eyelashes should feel comfortable. Start full eyelash strips here, not too close to the inner corner of the eye.**

## Individual False Eyelashes

If you are simply looking to enhance your natural look, I prefer individual lashes. Keep in mind, though, that they take longer to apply than strips. First, I gently curl natural lashes and apply mascara. Next I dip the base of the false eyelashes into eyelash glue, using tweezers, careful only to get a small amount of glue on the base. I allow the glue to dry for a few seconds to make it more adhesive, then I place the base of the lashes close to the lash line, paying attention to any gaps there may be in the lash line. Doing it in this order gives false lashes the now curled natural lashes to balance on. Otherwise, the lash usually falls into the eyes.

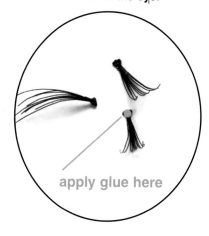

**apply glue here**

## Full Strip False Eyelashes

Strips are great for dramatic looks or for eyes that have very sparse lashes or a flat lid with no crease. I also love them for period looks. You can make strip lashes appear more natural by getting some with hairs that vary in length (see photo).

You can do full strips in two different ways depending on your preference. You can gently curl eyelashes first, apply mascara, then apply glue along the base of the strip. Allow the glue to get tacky for a few seconds, then balance the strip on top of eyelashes, attaching false lashes as close to the lash line as possible. (If necessary use a pointy cotton swab to push lashes closer to the base.) Curling first will give the false lashes something to lie on so you don't have to hold them in place. Your other option is to curl your lashes after you have already applied the false lashes. This will allow the fake and existing lashes to blend together. There are pros and cons to both techniques as you'll notice. With both techniques, use black liquid eyeliner if necessary to darken the glue line after the glue has dried.

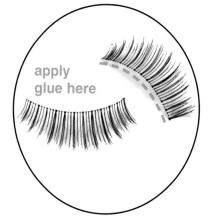

**apply glue here**

**Notice the differentiation in length on this lash strip, which gives a natural effect that is similar to the way real lashes grow.**

False eyelashes are something I think most women, Asian or not, are afraid of trying. I've definitely coerced many women into trying them for the first time whether they were young adults or in their seventies. You can make them look natural or dramatic. It depends on the type you choose.

## Full strip lashes

Full strips come in many forms (the set shown here is medium height and fullness). The longer and fuller they are the more dramatic effect they'll add to your eyes. For a natural look, avoid glittery or very dense lashes.

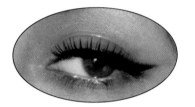

### Three-quarter strip lashes

These lashes are hard to find, but look amazing. Notice how they crisscross at the base as natural lashes would. I love these because they'll never poke you in the inner corners of the eye even if you put them on wrong.

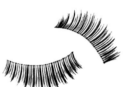

### Individual lashes

Individual lashes create the most natural look. You can't even tell they're there most of the time. They are difficult to apply if you have minimal lashes, though, so stick with three-quarter length or full lashes if that's the case.

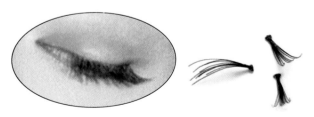

## Lower lashes

I usually only use lower lashes for strong period looks like the 1960s look shown here. I have been known to wear them out at night, but always with smoky eye makeup and always with upper lashes as well. If you have minimal lashes lay them on top of your existing lashes; otherwise apply them beneath your lower lashes.

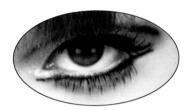

I've heard many times from Asian women that they simply don't bother with their lashes because they have so few lashes they don't see the point. The reality is even if your lashes seem sparse, there are many products you can use to make your lashes look fuller, giving your eyes a more open, youthful look.

### Mascara

When purchasing mascara look for products with small brushes with defined bristles that'll separate and are not too wet (a good way to test this is if there is a big clump on the mascara brush and the liquid looks somewhat drippy). Heavy mascaras will make natural lashes fall. Waterproof mascara is a great option for Asian women who have trouble with lashes staying up. It will also help lashes hold curl longer and is easy to take off if you have a great eye makeup remover. Look for silicone-based eye makeup removers that remove mascara easily.

### Lash curler

You definitely get what you pay for with lash curlers. My favorites are high-end metal lash curlers that are usually made in Japan and found in department stores. You'll notice that you only need one squeeze to curl Asian lashes—this is not the case with drugstore brands yet. For natural-looking lashes, curl at the base, middle, and tips of eyelashes.

## Lash glue

Yes, you even have to be careful in choosing your lash glue. Make sure that the glue is not too runny or too strong. If the glue is too strong the lashes can be very painful to take off, which is terrible for the delicate eyelid area. The very strong glues tend to be clear and you can feel the fumes when the glue gets close to your eyes. I prefer glue in a tube that comes out white and dries clear, usually a latex base.

## Lash extensions

Lash extensions are expensive and high-maintenance, but if you're that type of girl they may be worth the cost. Extensions are conceptually a brilliant idea and are great if you don't wear eye makeup daily and have the money and time for upkeep. Hairs are glued onto existing hairs. They have to be attached to natural hairs so if you don't have many it may not be worth it for you. This must be done by a professional who has been specifically trained to do lash extensions. The extensions can be attached to both upper and lower lids. I've seen lash extensions look so natural that I couldn't tell where the real lashes began and extensions ended. Extensions take a few hours to apply and last one to two months and touch-ups have to be done in between, usually after two weeks for any hairs that may have fallen off. I, however, recommend every week. If they don't get touched up the hairs twist around and can't be pulled off manually. You also can't use certain makeup products with extensions, usually any makeup that contains any form of oil, cream shadows, some liners, and no mascara. When applying liner and shadows, it becomes a little more difficult as you have to constantly be careful while working around the lashes.

## Lash tinting

You have to get this done at a reputable salon as it can be very dangerous if you use the wrong dye and you could even be blinded. Tinting colors the lashes but doesn't add bulk. I personally didn't notice much difference when I got mine tinted as my lashes are black anyway, but women with paler or full lashes might find it appealing.

## Lash perming

Think of this as similar to a regular perm. Lashes are wrapped around small rods to curl them up. I notice very little difference in results between this and an eyelash curler. In fact, I think a metal eyelash curler works a thousand times better. Call me old school, but I prefer mascara and an eyelash curler.

## False individual lashes

False individual lashes have three to four single hairs attached to one tip. They are great for women who have some lashes and only want to fill in gaps or just need some lashes at the ends to lift or lengthen the eye.

## Single lashes

I hardly ever use these myself because they are harder to use and take a long time to apply. Single lashes are literally individual hairs that are applied to the lash line. You can use these for a truly separated lash look, but they do fall more often on Asian eyes as they don't have many natural hairs to sit on. I use a strong glue with these because they do fall so quickly.

## False lash strips

I think a lot of women say they have tried strips and found them too fake looking. However, strips are very versatile and come in dozens of different styles. Some will give you a retro look while others will give you a winged eye (see page 52). When looking for strips pay attention to the shape of your eye. If you have narrow, wide-set eyes, look for lashes that will open up your eyes, drawing lashes up not farther out. This means lashes that have length in the center of the strip and taper down at both ends. If your eyes are more close-set, choose lashes that start short and have length at the ends of the lashes. This draws eyes out. When in doubt try a few different styles to see what's best for you. You never learn unless you try—and have some fun with them!

**Cool Tip**
Without glue, first measure strips to the length of your eye, remove and cut at the ends where necessary, then follow application directions.

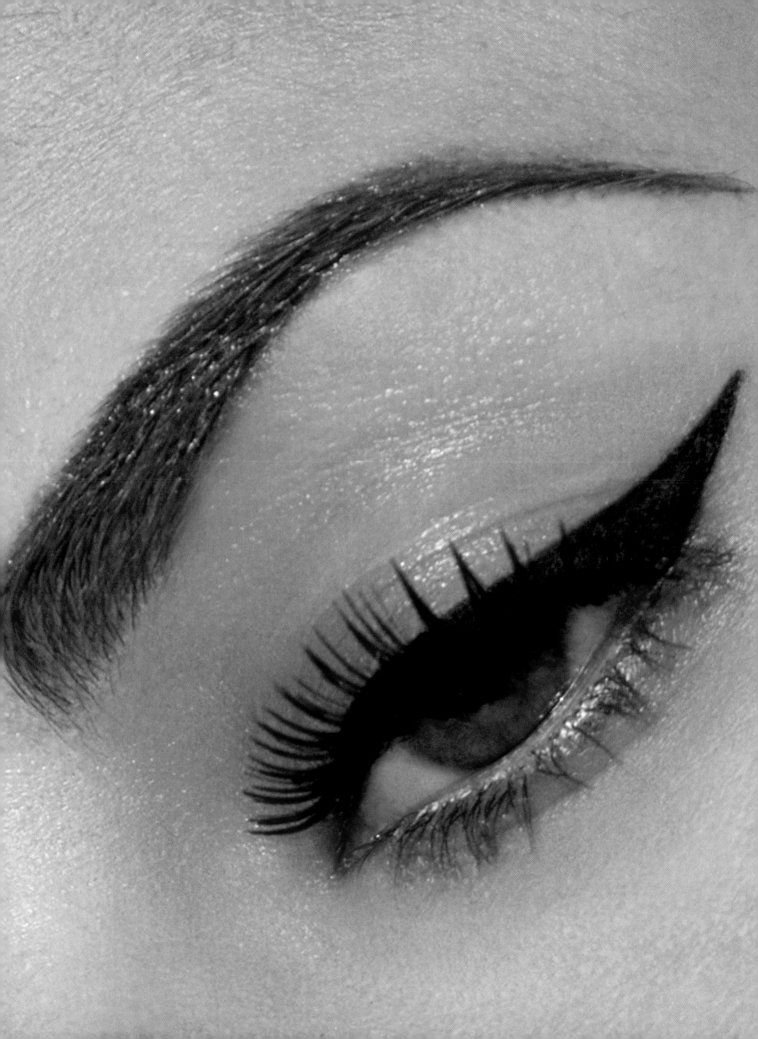

# eyeliner

Eyeliner is definitely one of the harder cosmetics to apply. However, like everything else in life, the harder you work at it, the better the results. Eyeliner can make the difference between the illusion of a large or small eye, and a sexy or plain eye. Back in the day there were not many choices for eyeliner. Liquid liners were too runny and pencils were hard and painful to work with. The way I kept eyeliner on when I was younger was to burn an eyeliner pencil and wait for it to cool slightly before applying it. There was more than one incident where I was in a hurry and burned myself. You should never do anything similar, not only because it's incredibly dangerous but because it's unnecessary. Today's eyeliners have definitely come a long way.

## Eyeliner at Work

The use of eyeliner can completely change the shape of your eye. On Emily, I used only a hint of eyeliner. For Meiling's looks, I used a much larger amount. For look 1, I extended the eyes using black liner to give her a modern punk look. For look 2, I used a heavier line of black eyeliner and smudged it into layer 3. This gives her a sexy, smoky look and creates the illusion of much larger eyes.

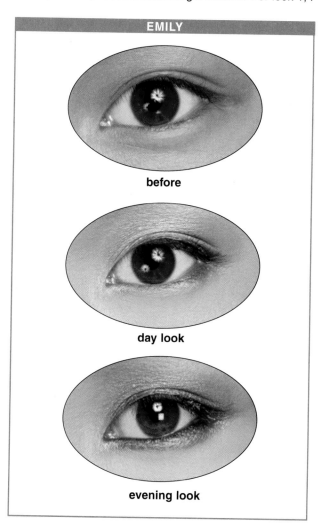

**EMILY**

before

day look

evening look

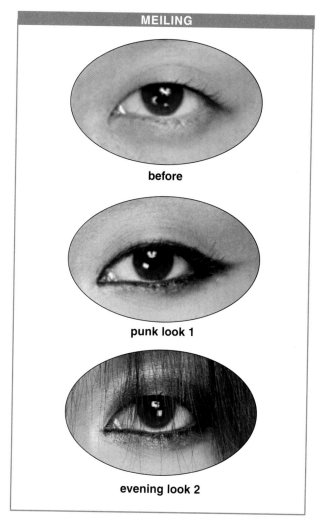

**MEILING**

before

punk look 1

evening look 2

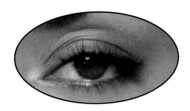

## Natural

This look is achieved by adding a little liner at the ends of the eyes to create a soft daytime look.

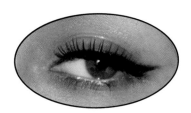

## Winged eye

Notice how the liner is applied in this look. White liner is applied inside the lower rim and a thick line of liquid liner on top gives Shazia a completely different look.

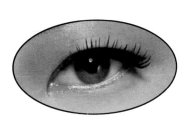

## Top lid

This is probably my favorite technique for a natural look that is still defined. The eye looks finished while still looking fresh and clean. Apply a thin line of your favorite black eyeliner on the top lid as close to the lash line as possible. I applied a white liner in the lower rim to achieve this look (optional).

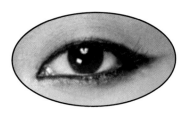

## Punk

Great for the adventurous girl or for costume looks. Putting liner on top and bottom lids and extending past the ends of the eye really adds length to the eye. You can do a less extreme version of this just to add length, which I do often with my smoky looks.

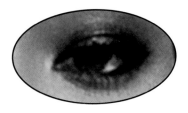

## Smoky

I love this look and it's probably one most Asian women don't attempt because they are unsure how to achieve it. Use a liner brush to smudge liner out. Pair it with a nude or neutral lip.

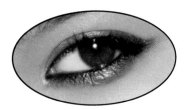

## Colored cream liner

This liner comes in so many colors now from bright pinks to metallic charcoal grays. I often use it instead of eye shadow to create a more clean smoky eye. (Paired here with black eyeliner.)

## Gel liner

This is one of the newcomers to the eyeliner world. I had to get used to the idea of working with a gel liner because I, like everyone else in the makeup business, was skeptical, but now I can't live without it. It's a great tool to create a perfect sharp line and is also great for mature skin. It gives the eye a lined look without pulling at the delicate skin! You do need to work quickly, as once it's set it doesn't move.

## Liquid liner brush

Liquid eyeliner is almost always found in a tube similar to mascara and comes with its own brush. If you are a novice to liquid eyeliners look for a stiff applicator made of a dense synthetic material. Glide the tip of the brush along the outer lash line, pressing lightly for a thin line and increasing pressure for a thicker line.

## Liquid liner foam

I like this dense foam liner because it's more forgiving than a brush and gives you the control of a pencil, without losing the sharp liquid liner look.

## Eyeliner pencil

You get what you pay for when it comes to pencil eyeliner. Avoid pencil liners that are waxy and hard, as they pull at the skin and don't deposit enough color. Pencils should be soft and go on smoothly. I love eyeliner pencils because I can smudge the line I draw with an eyeliner brush and create a sultry, smoky eye. Set this liner with shadow to minimize bleeding and use waterproof liner for defined lines that don't smudge or smear. Pencils are especially great for lower lids.

**Cool Tip**

Use liquid liner to cover eyelash glue and to redarken lashes that already have mascara on them. It makes lashes dark again without the added clumping that comes from applying a second coat of mascara.

## Waterproof liner

Most eyeliners of any type are available in waterproof form, which is great for Asian women because, due to the shape of some Asian eyelids, liners tend to smudge, particularly on the lower lids. If you are investing in a waterproof liner, definitely splurge on one that goes on smoothly and doesn't pull at the skin around the eye.

## Colored cream liners

Consider colors other than black or brown. I love to use colored liners in layer 3 (see page 43) instead of shadow for a long-lasting intense eye. They are a little heavier than cream shadows so they last longer, and come in nice shimmers as well. If you're using a fun color make sure you add black or brown liner in layer 4 to help neutralize the look. With colored liners look for creamy textures that don't crumble and aren't too waxy or hard in texture. If it glides on smoothly and stays put, you have a winner. If you really have a smudging problem you can also use gel liners.

**Cool Tip**

Make sure you always sharpen the tips of liners so they are completely clean before each use. And never share eye makeup as you risk infection.

## White liner

Use white liner to mark off your brow tweezing area (see page 33). Look for one with a creamy texture. You can get away with using an inexpensive brand for this purpose. White liner that has beige tones is also great to use on the lower rim of the eye to brighten and open up tired red eyes (see page 69). Pure white liner should only be used for a dramatic or costume look.

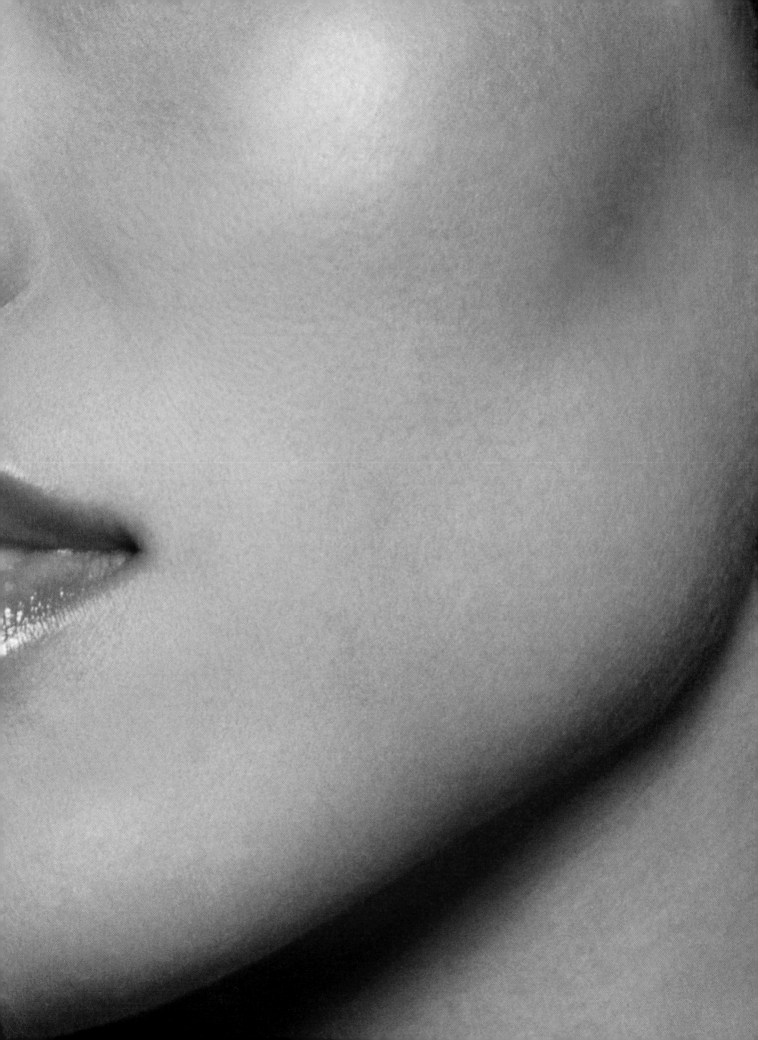

As a general guideline, keep the cheeks minimal for a more natural look, so that the focus will be on other areas like the lips or eyes. When applying blush, you should try to replicate your cheeks' color when slightly flushed. I prefer pale shimmery pinks and apricots as well as corals and berries for very dark skin.

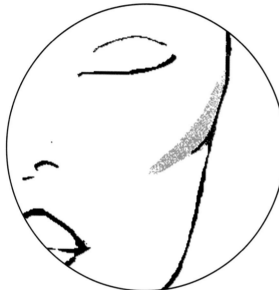

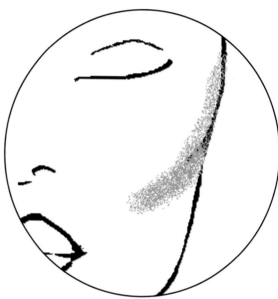

Apply blush just under the cheekbone to accentuate the line of the cheekbone.

For rounder faces apply blush closer to the nose.

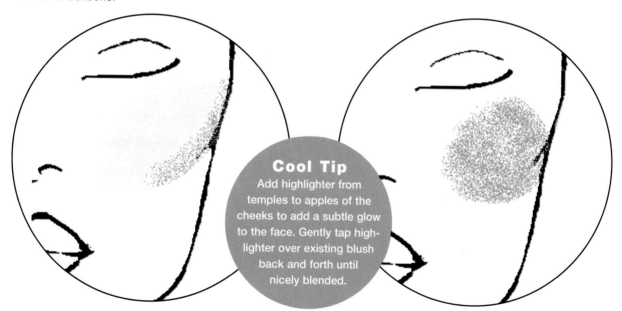

**Cool Tip**
Add highlighter from temples to apples of the cheeks to add a subtle glow to the face. Gently tap highlighter over existing blush back and forth until nicely blended.

Here is my favorite way to apply blush: Use a darker contour color below the cheekbones to emphasize the cheekbones and a subtle color on the apples of the cheeks for a soft blend. This adds dimension and color without appearing too harsh.

Apply blush to the apples of the cheeks. Apply heavily to give you a strong china-doll look or more subtly to add an instant youthfulness to your face.

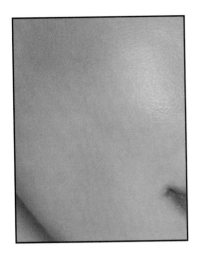

## Contour + shimmery blush on the apples

This is probably my favorite look. The contoured cheek still looks soft and pretty when paired with a soft peach or pink color on the apples of the cheeks.

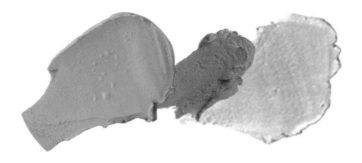

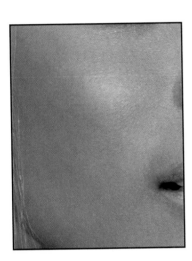

## Bronzer

I love using bronzer, especially during the spring and summer, to create sexy, dramatic looks. If you have pale skin, stick with a very soft, sheer, light brown bronzer only one or two shades darker than your natural skin tone.

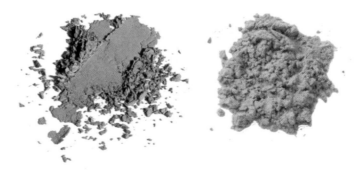

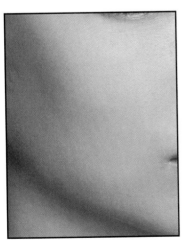

## Natural and matte

Use a little blush on the apples or along the cheekbones to give a soft, natural, understated look. My favorite is a warm pink.

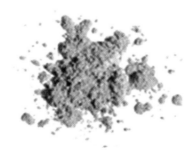

I didn't wear blush until I became very educated about it. When I was growing up in the '80s, the popular way to wear blush was in very strong, bright colors. That style has definitely changed. When it comes to blush, less is more. Your choice may be based on the look you are trying to achieve or even what kind of weather conditions you are dealing with. Here are some guidelines to the different types of blush.

## Cream blush

Cream blush comes in tubes and pots and ranges from dry to a little glossy. This is a great choice if you have dry or mature skin and want more of a youthful glow. Easy to blend, the blush is best applied starting with a small amount on the apples and blending toward the temples, working in downward and outward (toward temples) swipes. Use a wedge sponge to clean up any excess.

## Blush stain

Blush stain is great for hotter weather or if you have a tendency to sweat. Apply to clean, moisturized skin. (This allows better blending.) If you're wearing foundation, apply stain after foundation and before powder. Sometimes stains are hard to remove. If you've used too much and need to make some adjustments, use makeup remover. If it still hasn't completely come off, use foundation or concealer to cover the area (this will help subdue the color).

## Liquid highlighter

Liquid highlighter is perfect to use on the area above the apples of the cheeks near the temples. It gives the cheeks that glow you see in magazine spreads. It's quite easy to achieve this look as it's all about using the right product. Look for products whose descriptions contain key words like "highlighter" or "illuminating." To apply, place a little bit of the product on your finger and dab along the top part of the cheekbone.

## Gel blush

Gel blush looks like Jell-O and is similar to a blush stain but easier to work with, as it is not as intense in color as the stain, but lasts almost as long.

## Powder blush

Powder blush is an oldie but a goodie. Powder is great for women of all ages. It comes in every color under the sun and in all kinds of textures. I prefer powders that have a tiny bit of shimmer in them, creating a soft, pearly hue.

### Cool Tip
To make blush last longer use a tiny amount of cream blush as your base coat and finish with a powder blush.

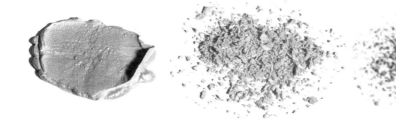

# contouring

Contouring can be a very scary thought for most women because I think the normal perception is that contouring involves drawing dark lines at the sides of the nose or harsh cheekbone lines. Contouring actually eliminates the white-face look that I see so many Asian women do. I contour almost every face that I see because most women have different color skin tone on their faces than they do their chest or arms. When contouring it's important to keep the highlight and contour colors only a shade or two apart from one another to create a natural look.

Blending is key to contouring. The center of the face should always be lighter than the outer parts (forehead, jawline, cheekbone) of the face. It's important to blend the two shades lightly together so there are no harsh lines separating the shade. However, this doesn't mean that you should mix the two shades completely. Instead, make sure to blend only the outer edges of each shade to connect the two colors together gently.

## Light Contouring

Once you've found your favorite foundation I recommend buying another foundation one shade lighter or darker than that color. Most skin colors do change a shade throughout the year (see page 17).

## Heavy Contouring

If I want to make a person's skin look significantly lighter, darker, or more sculpted (see page 123), I use cream or stick foundations as they offer heavier coverage and hide natural skin tones better than other types of foundation.

## For Very Dark Skin

Many women with dark skin already have a bit of natural contouring because their skin tone often varies across their face. It's more important to contour dark skin because it's more likely to have strong contrast in color from the center of the face (bottom of forehead, under eyes, chin, and nose) to the outside of the face (top of the forehead, jawline, and cheekbones). If you were to test makeup on your jawline (as someone with light skin would) and use the matching jawline color all over your face, you would realize that you now look much darker than you did without makeup. This is because many times the outer parts of your face may be dark with red undertones and the center of your face will be several shades lighter with yellow undertones. Contouring using those colors is essential to get the perfect foundation match. If you are a makeup novice, it might be wise to go to the makeup counter and find an artist with similar coloring to yours, whose makeup look you admire. If you are more than two shades different on your forehead than under your eyes you might have to get two different powders as well—one for the center of your face, the other for the outside of your face. If you can only purchase one, get the lighter tone and make sure it's sheer (see page 60).

# Contouring Using Powder
**(You can also use foundation in their different forms.)**

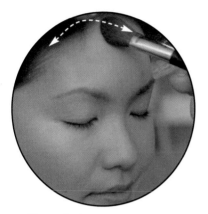

## To minimize a larger forehead

Use a contour shade here to minimize the forehead or darken the appearance of the face to match your body's skin tone.

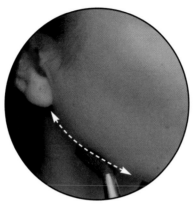

## Contour mature skin

Apply contour shade from under the earlobe along the jawline to the chin.

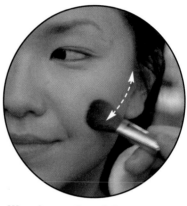

## Illusion of a thinner face or higher cheekbones

Apply contour shade from under the temple along the underside of the cheekbone and stop directly under the center of the apple of your cheek. For an already thin face, end the stroke earlier or extend the stroke closer to the nose for an even thinner effect.

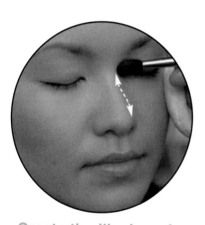

## Create the illusion of a bridge of the nose or thin out your nose

Apply straight lines along the sides of the nose. The area that is not shadowed will determine the width of the nose you create. Move the lines closer to the center of the nose for an even thinner effect. (For a natural effect highlight the bridge using a lighter foundation only.)

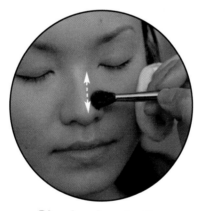

## Shadowing to the ball of the nose

Shadow the sides of the ball of the nose as well to continue a thinner nose. If the area is already thin, this step is unnecessary, but I've found that most people do require this step as well.

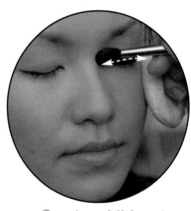

## Create additional depth to the eyelids

Brush on contour shade from the lash line to the middle of the eyelid.

# lightening skin

It has been embedded in some Asian cultures that lighter skin is more regal and is placed in high regard. I find beauty in all skin tones and disagree with this completely. However, I've seen too many pink-faced Asians, trying to be lighter than their natural tone, to ignore this practice. Another time you may need to lighten skin is if you've ignored sunscreen and your face is now too many shades darker than your body.

**To lighten skin, use your natural neck color as the contour shade and use one or two shades lighter than your natural skin tone for the high-light areas. This gives the appearance of lighter skin, but without the harsh separation of a light face and a dark neck that I see on so many women. Use your neck as a guide for outer color.**

**Natural skin color here is used as the contour shade.**

**Highlight color one or two shades lighter than natural skin tone.**

**Cool Tip**
Tap highlight and contour colors together at their edges to blend them.

# darkening skin

Although this completely disregards the cultural desire for lighter skin, I love creating beautiful golden skin. Especially when you live in warmer areas or like outdoor activities. Many times using sunscreen can cause your face to be several shades lighter than your body. In such cases use this as your guide to darken your face while still looking natural.

**To darken skin, mix the highlight and contour colors on the neck (use the color of your chest as a guide). Then use the contour color on the outside of the face and highlight colors in the center of the face. If your chest is much darker than your neck, don't mix the colors on the neck; instead, apply only the contour color (chest color) and continue contouring the face.**

Natural skin color here is used as the shade.

Contour color one to two shades darker than natural skin tone.

**Cool Tip**
Choosing contour colors that are too dark can make your skin look dirty.

**Cool Tip**
Use a synthetic foundation brush to get a cleaner application.

OVER THE PAST several years I've worked with many different types of women: homemakers, celebrities, teenagers, seventy-year-olds, underprivileged women, even presidents of billion-dollar companies. These women taught me a few things. One of the most important lessons I learned is just how much their desired looks varied. Often their day jobs dictated the type of makeup they wore.

Depending on whether you're a stay-at-home mom or a Hollywood celebrity, you are likely to have different ideas of what constitutes a daytime look. Comfort levels play a part as well. If you are not used to wearing makeup, a glamorous, smoky-eyed look is probably going to make you feel uncomfortable no matter how good it looks. This chapter contains several different looks for almost every daytime occasion. Try one and once you've mastered that, try them all. Most important, work with what you have. Asian women have come so far and I truly believe that you don't have to be pale and stick thin to be beautiful. Work with the shape and coloring you have, whether you're pale or dark, and you'll create a beautiful look. Drastic measures like plastic surgery and skin bleaching are not necessary to make you feel great about yourself.

# day faces

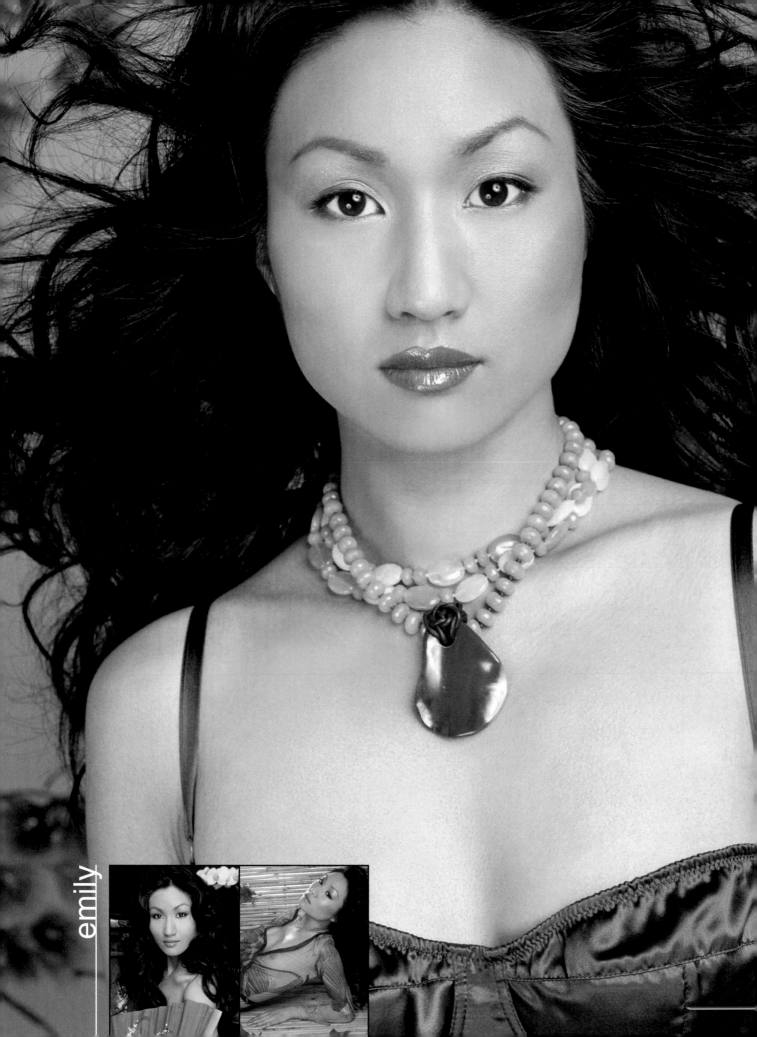

emily

1 Apply a highlight liquid foundation to the center of the face.
2 Blend in a contour liquid foundation to the outside of the face.
3 Apply under-eye cake concealer where necessary.
4 Use a darker cake concealer for the skin.
5 Set with translucent powder.
6 Apply brown brow pencil to brows.
7 Use a shimmery copper shadow at base and under eyes.
8 Blend a dark brown cream shadow in layer 3.
9 Apply black pencil eyeliner to top lid and lower corners.
10 Apply black waterproof mascara to top and bottom lids.
11 Apply bronzer along the cheekbones.
12 Apply cream highlighter above apples and at temples.
13 Line lips with warm brown lip liner.
14 Apply a copper lip gloss.
15 Apply bronzer all over neck and chest and shoulders.

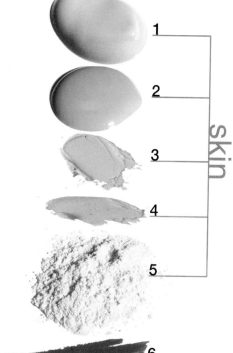

**skin** 1 2 3 4 5

## focal points

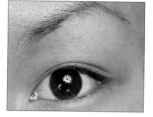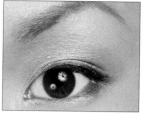

Apply **shimmery copper eye shadow** on lids (layer 2) and under the eyes to lighten and brighten eyes. I added a **brown cream shadow** at the base of the lid (layer 3) to add depth. **Black eyeliner** on the top lid and lower corners helps to bring the eyes up and out.

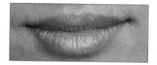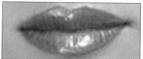

I used a **warm brown liner** to outline lips and put a few strokes in the center to avoid a dark outline. By slightly overdrawing Emily's upper lip I created a more symmetrical mouth. Fill in the outlined mouth with a **copper lip gloss**.

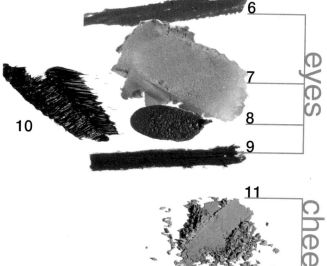

**eyes** 6 7 8 9 10

**cheeks** 11 12

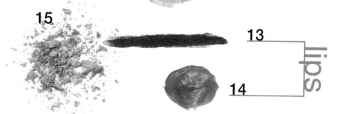

15

**lips** 13 14

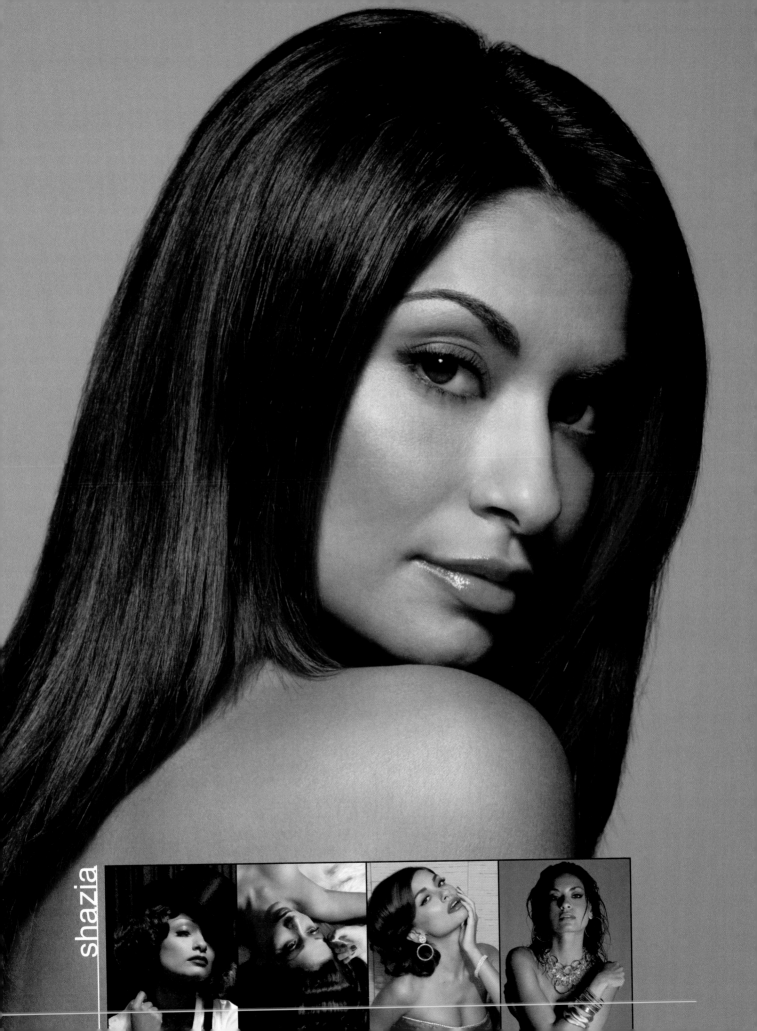

shazia

*I first met Shazia on a photo shoot and was impressed by her warm nature, humor, and style. You may recognize her from covers of magazines, as the music video "it" girl, or from her films. As one of Bollywood's rising stars, Shazia is not only beautiful, she also has a look that can change dramatically as you can see from her other photos.*

1 Apply a highlight foundation to the center of the face.
2 Blend in a contour foundation to the outside of the face.
3 Apply under-eye concealer where necessary.
4 Use a darker concealer for the skin.
5 Set with a golden loose powder.
6 Apply neutral brown brow cream to brows.
7 Use a neutral brown shadow at base.
8 Apply a taupe shadow on the brow bone.
9 Apply black eyeliner.
10 Apply black mascara.
11 Apply short black individual eyelashes.
12 Apply bronzer along the cheekbones.
13 Apply shimmery highlighter above apples and at temples.
14 Apply neutral lip liner.
15 Apply pale champagne lip gloss.
16 Apply clear lip gloss.

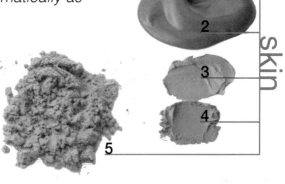

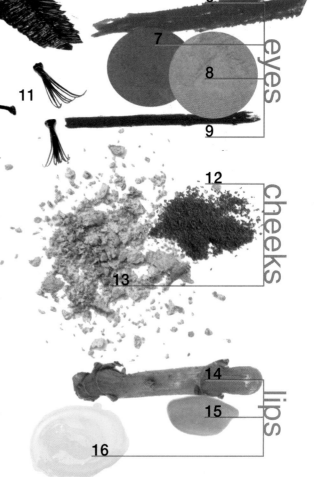

*skin*

*eyes*

*cheeks*

*lips*

## focal points

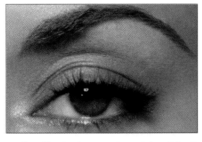

Use a **neutral brown shadow** over base of the lid. I used a **golden taupe color eye shadow** at the brow bone. Then line the top and bottom lash line with a **black eye pencil**. I finished off the look by curling the lashes and applying **black mascara** to the top and bottom lashes. Apply a few **short black individual lashes** on the outer corners.

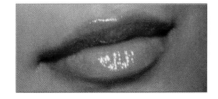

I applied a **neutral lip liner** and added a **champagne lip gloss**, topping it off with a **clear gloss** to add extra shine.

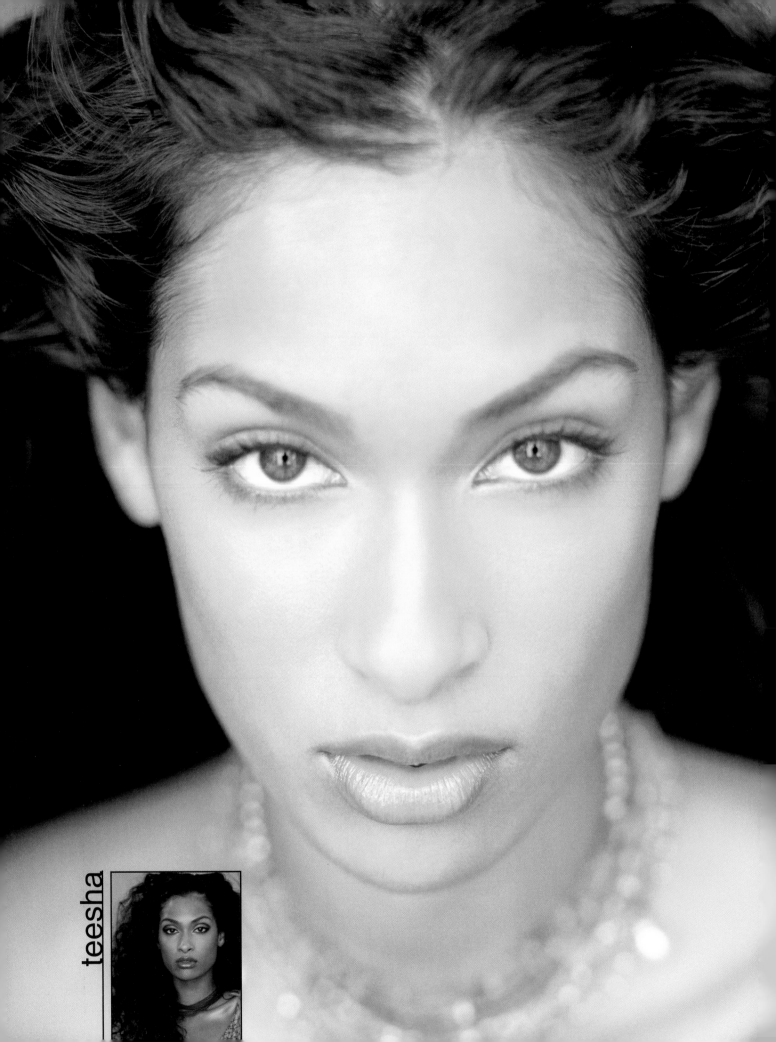

teesha

# summer breeze

1 Apply a highlight foundation to the center of the face.
2 Blend in a contour foundation to the outside of the face.
3 Set with golden brown loose powder.
4 Apply ash dark brown brow cream to brows.
5 Use a warm brown shadow at base of eyelid.
6 Apply a dark brown pencil liner close to lash line, then wing up at ends.
7 Apply a champagne highlighter cream pencil to the inner corners of the eyes.
8 Apply black mascara.
9 Apply coral blush to apples of cheeks.
10 Apply powder highlighter above apples and at temples.
11 Apply warm brown lip liner.
12 Apply warm coral lip gloss.

## focal points

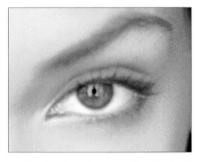

Use a **warm brown shadow** over base of the eyelid. Then line the top and bottom lash line using **dark brown eyeliner**. For the top lash line I winged the ends to give an uplifted look to the eyes. For the bottom I gently smudged the liner to create a softer look. I used a **champagne-colored cream highlighter eye pencil** on the inner corners of Teesha's eyes. Finish off the look with **black mascara** on the top and bottom lashes.

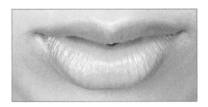

Teesha has beautiful large lips. I lined the top and bottom lips with a **warm brown lip liner**. Then I blended in a **warm coral lip gloss** to create a soft and pretty mouth.

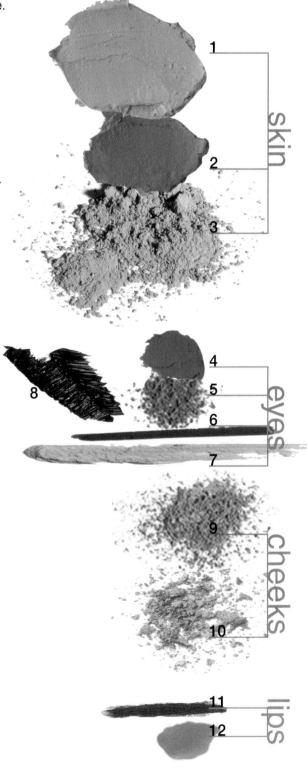

skin

eyes

cheeks

lips

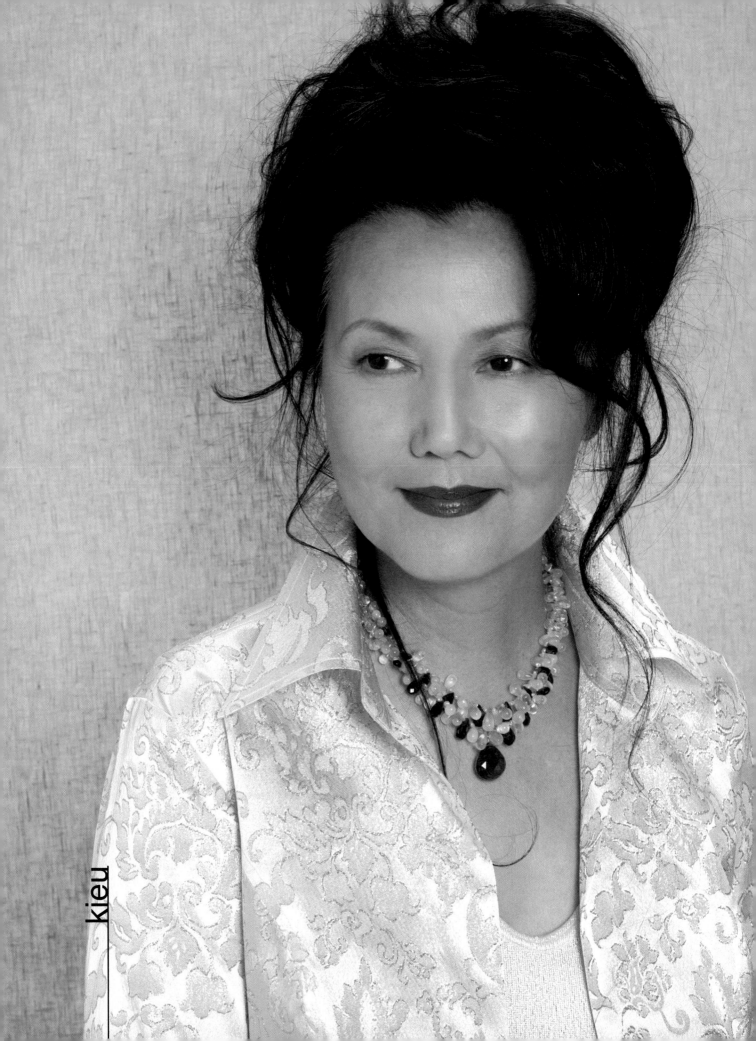

kieu

# beauty endured

*Kieu Chinh is an inspiration. She is one of the rare Asian women who has been on the small and big screen in Hollywood for decades and she's still going strong. She has helped tell so many touching stories with her presence. It was a true honor for me to glam her up in a way that she is rarely seen in front of the camera.*

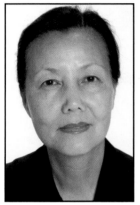

**kieu before**

1 Apply a highlight foundation to the center of the face.
2 Blend in a contour foundation to the outside of the face.
3 Apply under-eye concealer where necessary.
4 Use a darker concealer for the skin.
5 Set with translucent powder.
6 Apply brown brow pencil to brows.
7 Use a shimmery magenta shadow at base.
8 Apply black eyeliner.
9 Apply black mascara.
10 Apply blush along the cheekbones.
11 Apply a pink cream highlighter above apples.
12 Apply warm brown lip liner.
13 Apply dark magenta cream lipstick.

## focal points

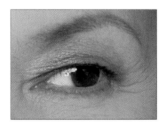

Use a **metallic magenta shadow** over the base of the eyelid and along the bottom lash line. I used **black eye pencil** on Kieu's lids and blended above to add symmetry to both eyes. I finished the look with **black mascara**.

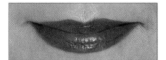

I applied a **warm brown lip liner** to create symmetry in Kieu's lips, adding a few jagged lines to the center so there is no line of demarcation. Then I blended in a **magenta cream lipstick** over the entire mouth.

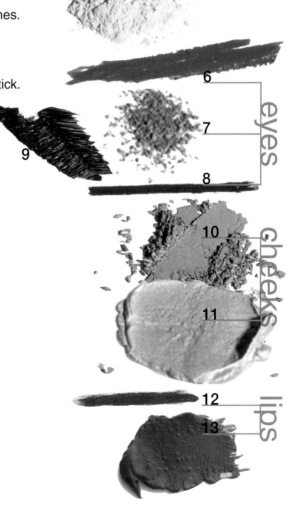

skin

eyes

cheeks

lips

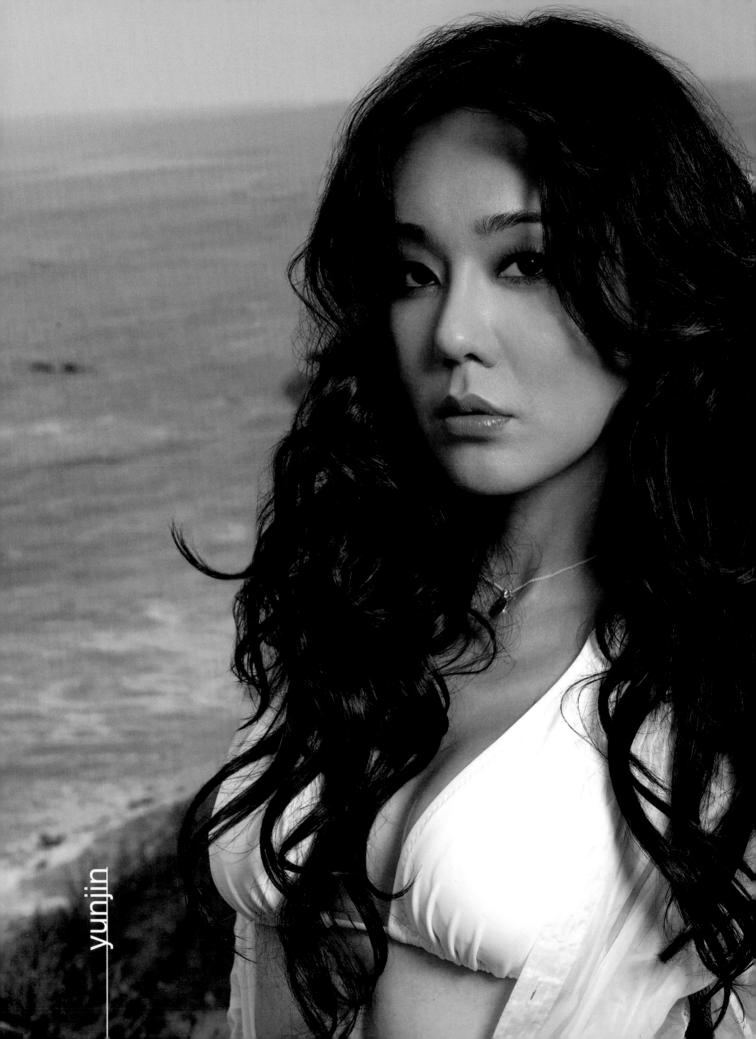

yunjin

# allure at sea

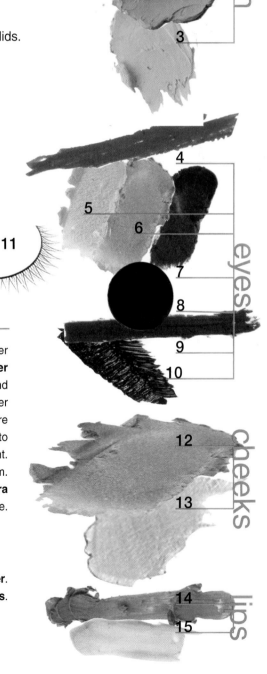

Yunjin Kim is an international superstar. An accomplished actress who made a name for herself in Korea and all over Asia, she is now making it in America on the hit TV series Lost. I was fortunate to meet her on a fashion cover shoot and was taken aback by her poise and elegance. Untainted by stardom she is humble and kind. Yunjin has a quiet strength about her that I find so alluring and incredibly beautiful.

1  Apply a stick foundation to the center of the face and on eyelids.
2  Blend in a contour foundation to the outside of the face.
3  Apply under-eye concealer where necessary.
4  Apply dark warm brown brow pencil to brows.
5  Use a cream gold highlighter under brow bone (layer 1).
6  Apply copper cream shadow at base (layer 2).
7  Blend in a dark brown cream shadow (layer 3).
8  Apply black eye shadow.
9  Apply black eyeliner.
10  Apply black mascara.
11  Apply full strip black eyelashes.
12  Apply cream bronzer along cheekbone.
13  Apply cream highlighter above apples and at temples.
14  Apply neutral lip liner.
15  Apply sheer pink lip gloss.

## focal points

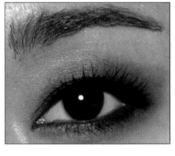

Use a **cream gold highlighter** under brow bone (layer 1). Apply **copper cream shadow** at base (layer 2). Blend in a **dark brown cream shadow** (layer 3). Apply **black eyeliner** around entire eye using a eyeliner blend brush to blend the top lid to desired height. Apply more black liner inside lower rim. Curl lashes and apply **black mascara** to the top and bottom lashes. Apply **full strip lashes** to the top lash line. Add **cream gold highlighter** to the inner corners.

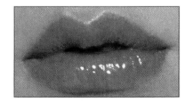

Softly line lips with a **neutral lip liner**. Finish with a **sheer baby pink lip gloss**.

skin

eyes

cheeks

lips

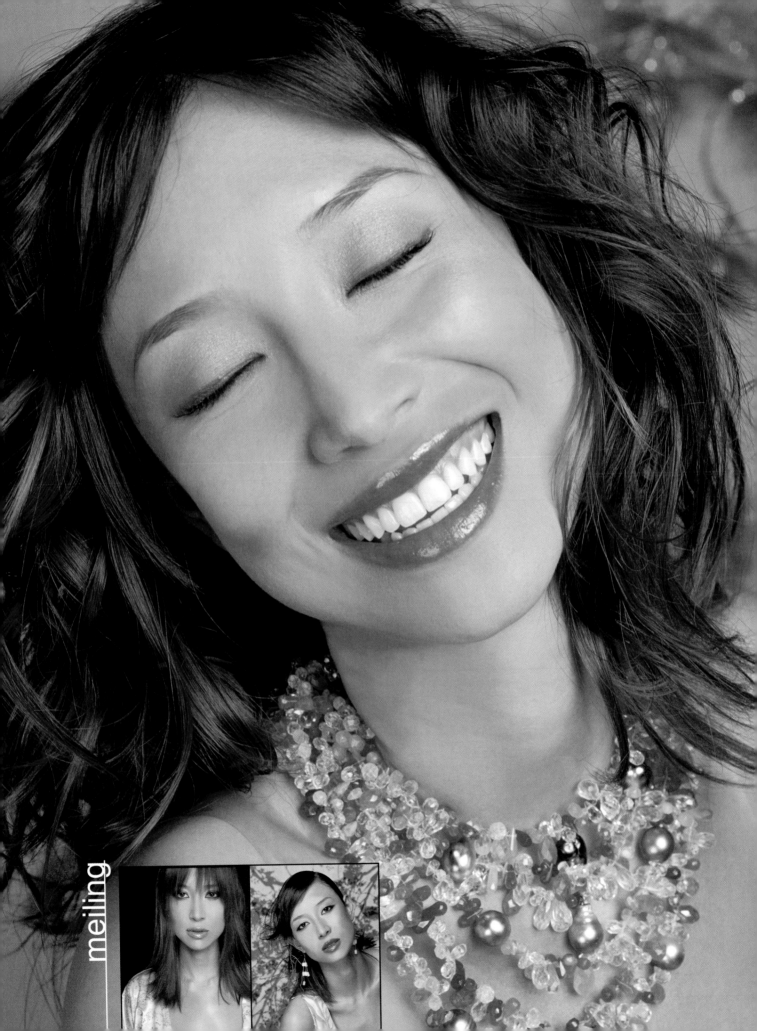

meiling

# the sweet life

*I was fortunate to meet Meiling on a photo shoot and then work with her on several more occasions and got to know her as a very skilled and fun-loving model and actress. You may have seen Meiling on the big screen or as a stunt double for some of the leading martial-arts actresses.*

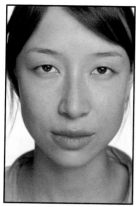

**meiling before**

1 Apply a highlight stick foundation to the center of the face.
2 Blend in a contour stick foundation to the out-side of the face.
3 Apply under-eye concealer where necessary.
4 Set with translucent yellow-based powder.
5 Apply ash brown brow cream to brows.
6 Apply shimmery rose-colored eye shadow.
7 Apply black eyeliner.
8 Apply black mascara.
9 Apply pink powder blush to apples of cheeks.
10 Apply cream highlighter above apples and at temples.
11 Apply neutral lip liner.
12 Apply dark rose-colored lip gloss.

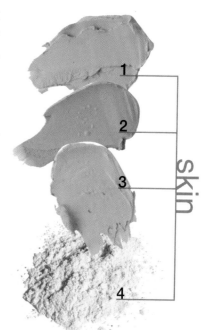

skin

## focal points

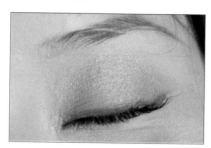

Use a **shimmery rose eye shadow** over base of the lid (layer 2). I used a **thick line of black eye pencil** on Meiling's lid and blended above the line to create a soft line to give definition to the lash line.

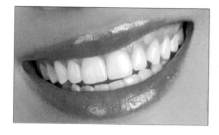

Meiling has beautiful large lips. I lined her lips with a **neutral lip liner** and blend-ed in a **dark rose lip gloss** over the entire mouth.

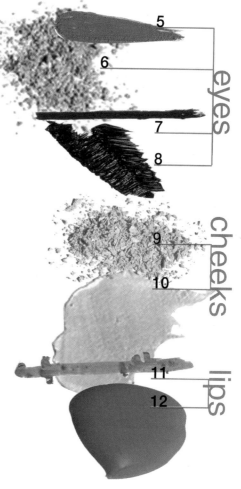

eyes

cheeks

lips

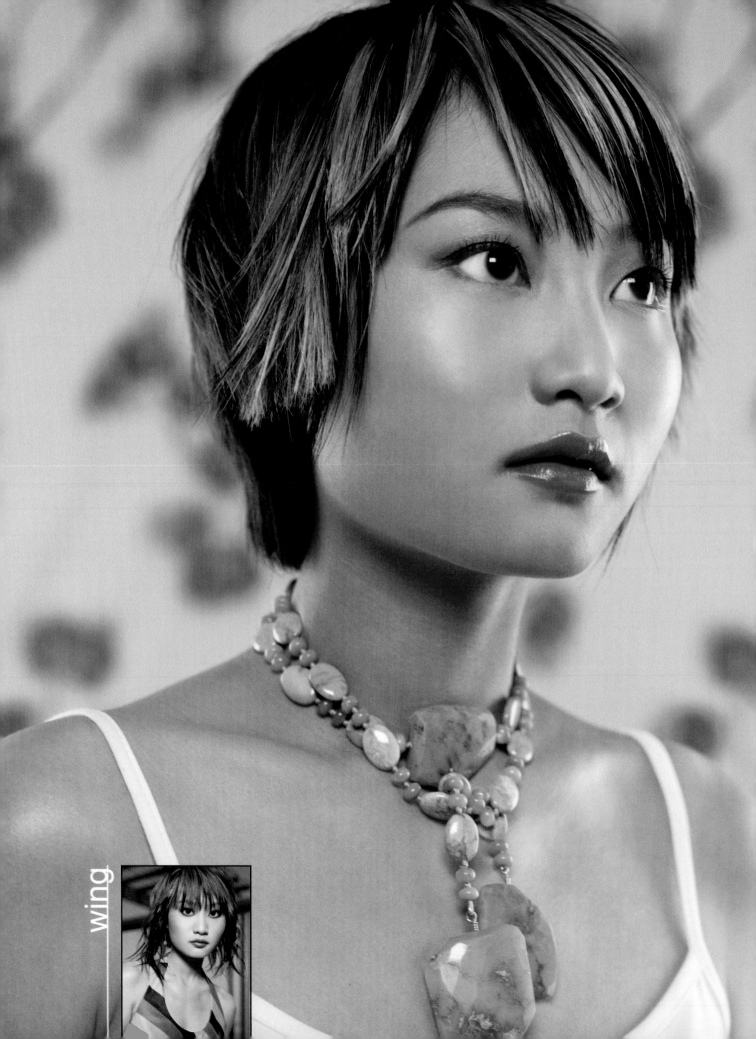

wing

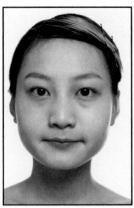

**wing before**

1 Apply a pearlized highlighter to the entire face and neck.
2 Apply a highlight cake foundation to the center of the face.
3 Blend in a contour cake foundation to the outside of the face.
4 Apply under-eye concealer where necessary.
5 Use a darker concealer for the skin.
6 Set with translucent yellow-based powder.
7 Apply ash brown brow cream to brows.
8 Use a lime green shadow at base.
9 Use soft green eye shadow in layer 3.
10 Apply black pencil eyeliner.
11 Apply black mascara.
12 Apply apricot blush to apples of cheeks.
13 Apply cream highlighter above apples and at temples.
14 Apply neutral lip liner.
15 Apply warm apricot lip gloss.

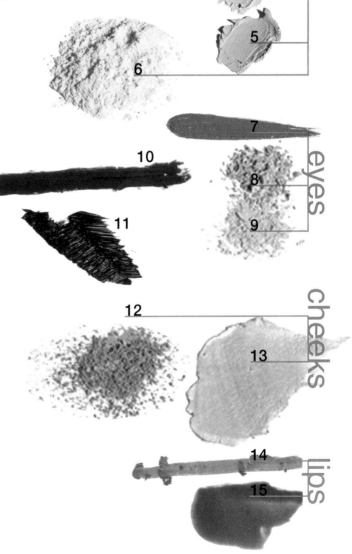

skin

eyes

cheeks

lips

## focal points

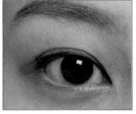

Use a **lime green eye shadow** over base of lid (layer 2). I used a **pale green shadow** on layer 3. I applied a thin line of **black eyeliner** along the top lash line. Curl lashes and finish the look with **black mascara** on top and bottom lashes.

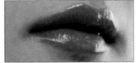

Wing has a smaller upper lip so I slightly overdrew the top using a **neutral lip liner**, lined the bottom lip along the natural lip line, added a few strokes of liner in the center, and blended in a **warm apricot lip gloss**.

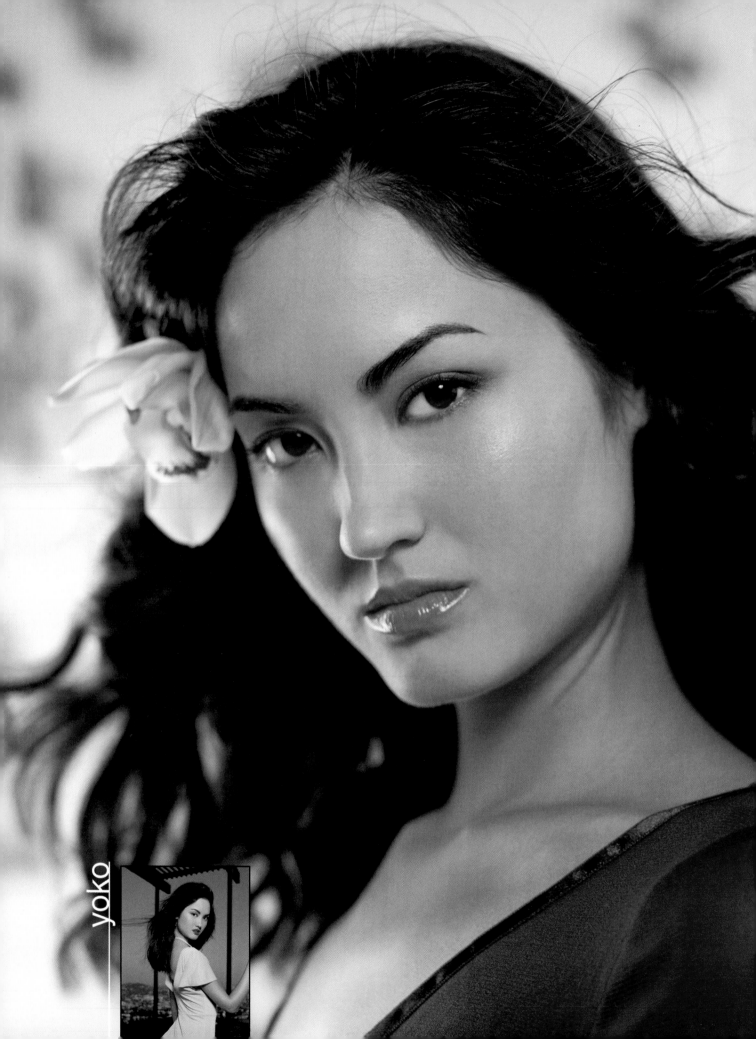

yoko

# lovely in lilac

1. Apply a pearlized highlighter to the entire face and neck.
2. Apply a highlight foundation to the center of the face.
3. Blend in a contour foundation to the outside of the face.
4. Apply under-eye concealer where necessary.
5. Set with translucent yellow-based powder.
6. Apply dark brown brow powder.
7. Use a shimmery wine eye shadow around entire eye.
8. Apply black eyeliner.
9. Apply black mascara.
10. Apply cream highlighter on apples of cheeks.
11. Apply neutral lip liner.
12. Apply grape and clear lip gloss.

## focal points

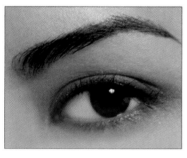

I used **dark brown brow powder** mainly on the ends of the brows to add soft definition to the eyebrow. Apply a **shimmery wine-colored eye shadow** around entire eye. I blended **black eyeliner** along the top and bottom lash line to add the illusion of fuller lashes. Curl lashes and add **black mascara** to top and bottom lashes.

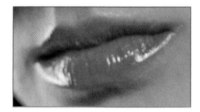

I mixed **grape and clear lip gloss** on Yoko's lips to give just a hint of color and a lot of shine.

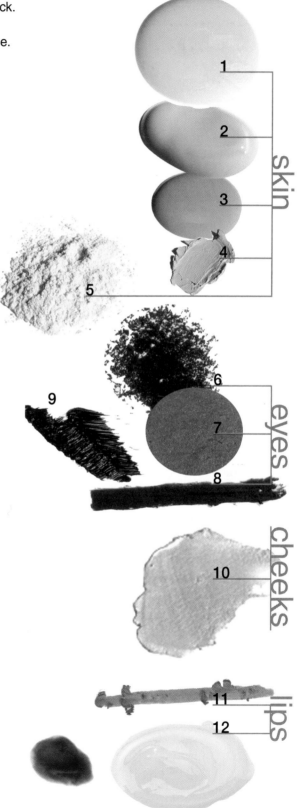

skin

eyes

cheeks

lips

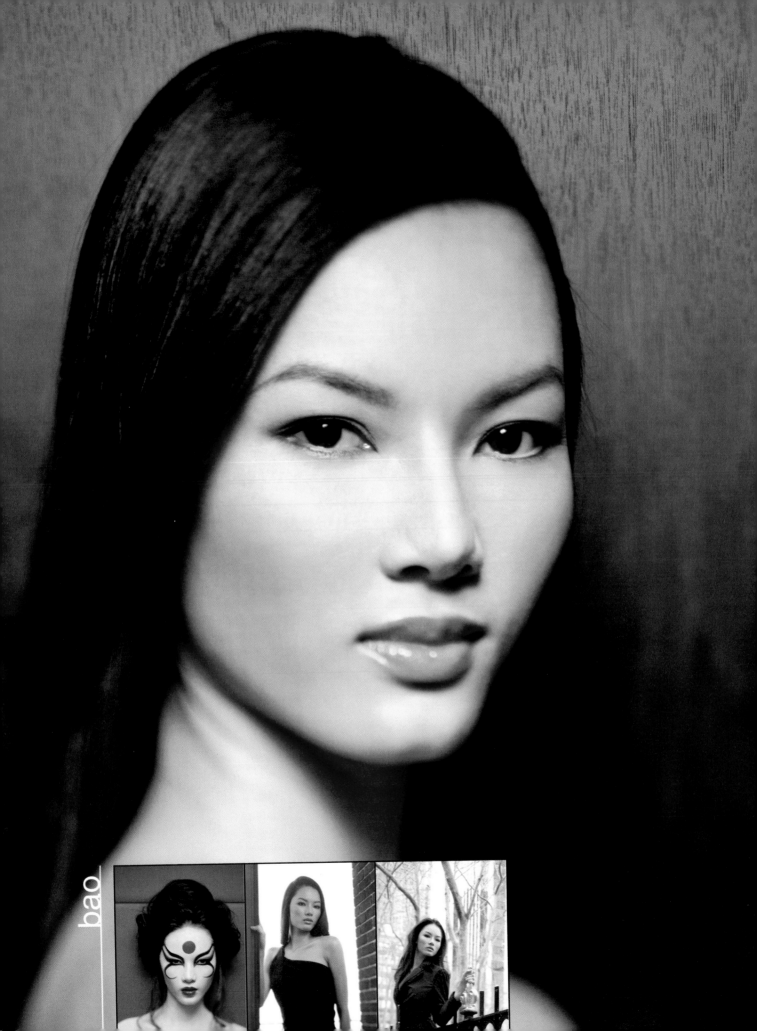

bao

1. Apply a highlight cream foundation to the center of the face.
2. Blend in a contour cream foundation to the outside of the face.
3. Apply under-eye concealer where necessary.
4. Set with translucent yellow-based powder.
5. Apply ash brown brow cream to brows.
6. Use a taupe eye shadow at base.
7. Use a chestnut eye shadow at lash line.
8. Apply black eyeliner.
9. Apply black mascara.
10. Apply pale bronzer along the cheekbone.
11. Apply cream highlighter above apples and at temples.
12. Apply neutral lip liner.
13. Apply beige and clear lip gloss.

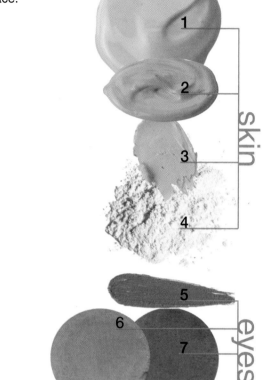

**skin**

## focal points

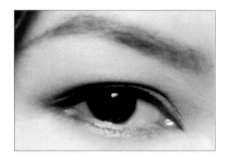

Use a **taupe brown shadow** over base of eyelid (layer 2). Apply **chestnut brown** in layer 3 to create depth to the eye. Also apply along lower lash line. Apply a thin line of **black eyeliner** along the top lash line.

Curl lashes and apply **black mascara** to top and bottom lashes.

**eyes**

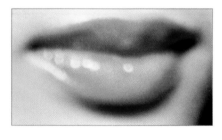

On Bao's lips I added definition to the natural lip line using a **neutral lip liner**, adding a few strokes to the center. Then I mixed **beige lip gloss** with clear to get a sheer look that allows some of the natural lip color to come through, giving Bao a pretty, natural look.

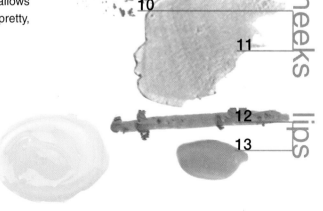

**cheeks**

**lips**

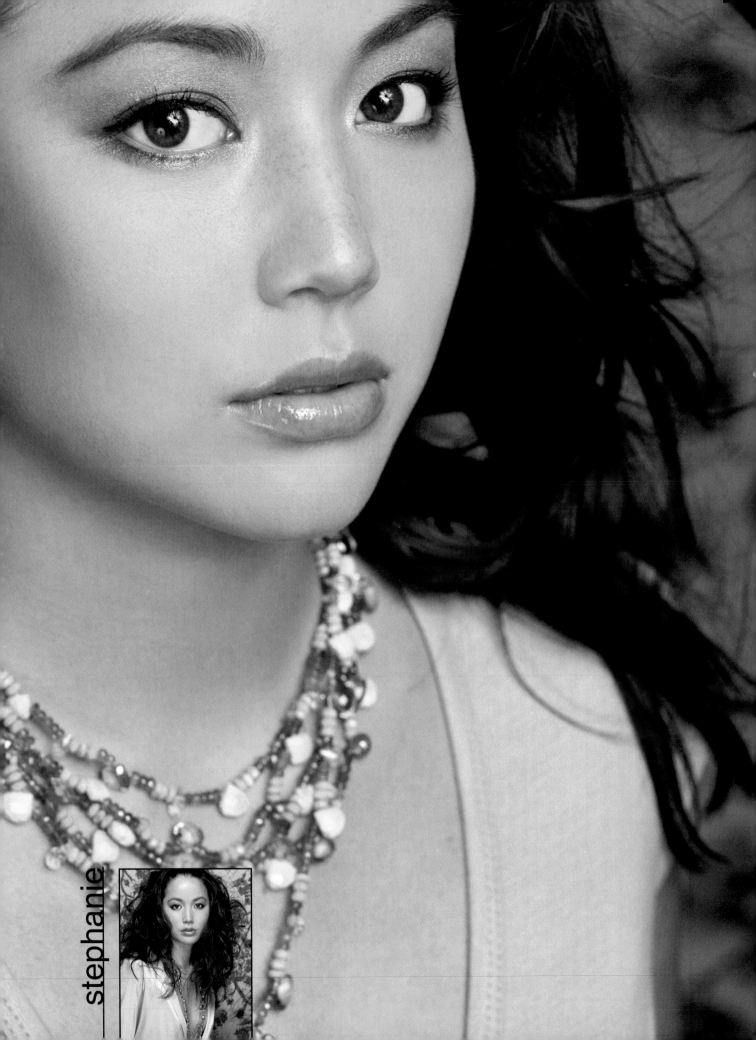

stephanie

1 Apply a highlight liquid foundation to the center of the face.
2 Blend in a contour liquid foundation to the outside of the face.
3 Set with translucent yellow-based powder.
4 Apply brown brow cream to brows.
5 Use a shimmery coral eye shadow at base.
6 Use shimmery plum on layer 3 and bottom lower corner.
7 Apply shimmery gold eye shadow to inner corner.
8 Apply black liquid eyeliner.
9 Apply black mascara.
10 Apply warm pink blush to apples of cheeks.
11 Apply neutral lip liner.
12 Apply sheer warm shimmery pink lip gloss.

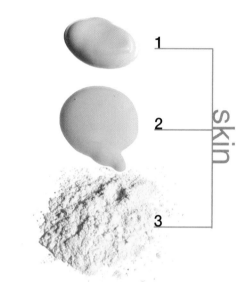

skin

## focal points

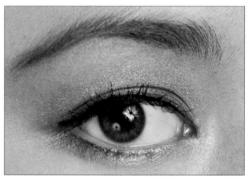

Use a **shimmery coral eye shadow** on the base of the lid. Apply a **shimmery plum shadow** on layer 3 and on the lower corners of the eyes. Apply **gold shimmery shadow** to the inner corners. Apply a thin line of **black eyeliner** to the top lash line and on the lower corner lash line. Curl lashes and apply **black mascara** to the top and bottom lashes.

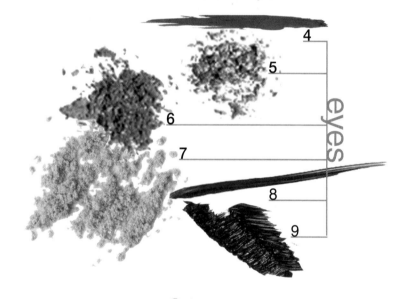

eyes

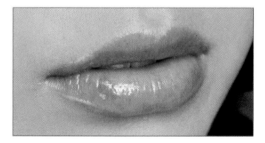

Apply **neutral lip liner** to define natural lip line. Blend a **shimery warm pink lip gloss** over entire mouth.

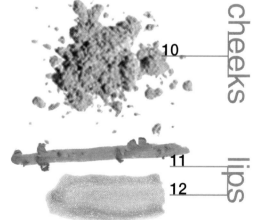

cheeks

lips

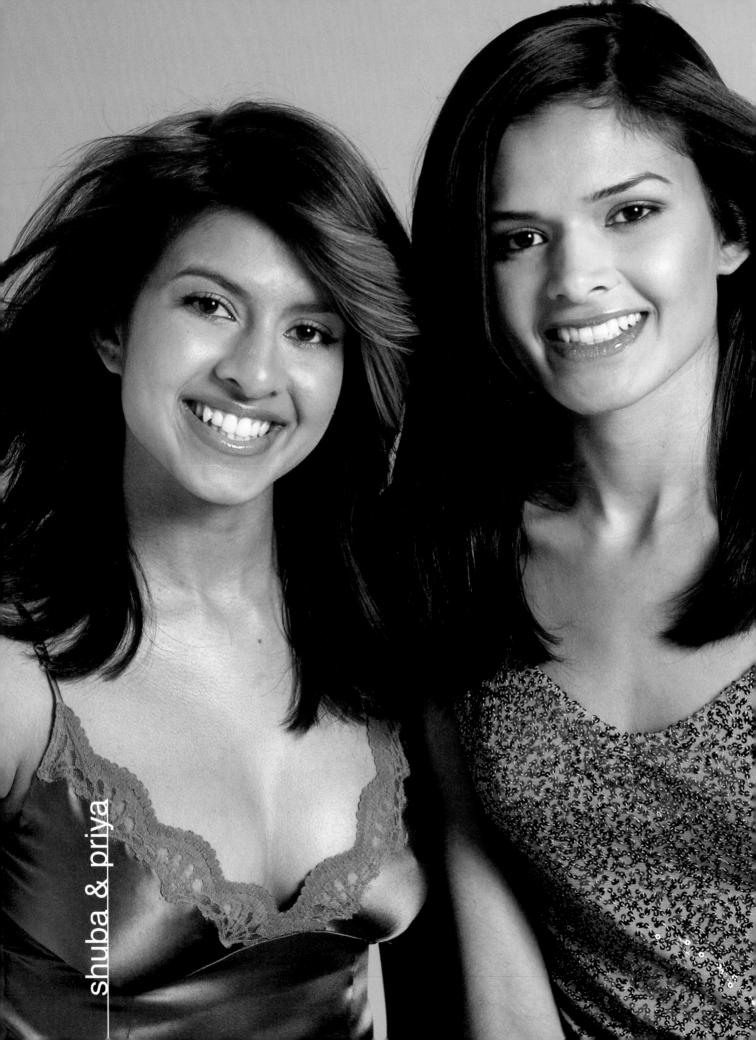

shuba & priya

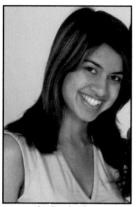

**shuba before**

1 Apply a highlight stick foundation to the center of the face.
2 Blend in a contour stick foundation to the outside of the face.
3 Apply under-eye concealer where necessary.
4 Use a darker concealer for the skin.
5 Set with a yellow-based pressed powder.
9 Apply black eyeliner inside lower rims and on top corners.
10 Apply black mascara.
11 Apply individual short black lashes.
12 Apply pink blush to apples of cheeks.
13 Apply cream highlighter above apples and at temples.

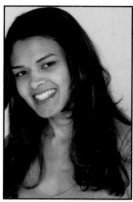

**priya before**

## focal points

6 Apply a **warm medium brown brow powder** to fill in brows and add definition to ends of brows. 7 Use a **pale salmon pink over base of lid and along bottom lash line**. 8 Apply shimmery pale beige eye shadow on brow bone and on center of eyelid and inner corner of the eye.

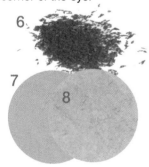

### what was the same

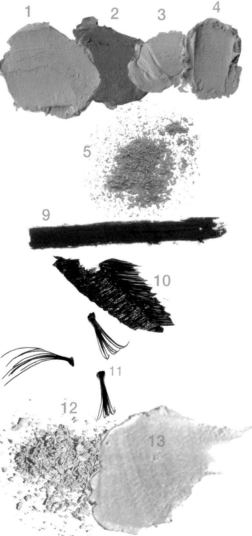

## focal points

6 Apply an **ashy brown brow pencil** to add definition to ends of brows. 7 Use a **plum eye shadow** over base of lid and along bottom lash line. 8 Apply **shimmery opal shadow** on brow bone and on center of eyelid and inner corner of the eye.

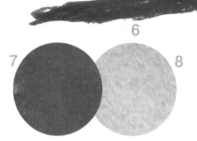

Apply **dark flesh lip liner** to define lips, then add a few strokes in center of lips. Apply a **pink creamy lipstick** over entire mouth. Finish with **clear gloss.**

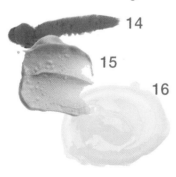

Apply **dark flesh lip liner** to define lips, then add a few strokes in center of lips. Apply a **warm pink shimmery lip gloss** over entire mouth.

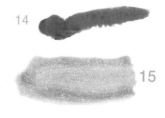

elaine & elisha

# mother and daughter

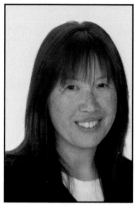

**elaine before**

1 Apply a highlight foundation to the center of the face. (Notice how it really evened out Elaine's skin tone but still looks natural.)

2 Blend in a contour foundation to the outside of the face (Elisha) and just along the cheekbone (Elaine).

3 Set with yellow-based pressed powder.

## what was the same

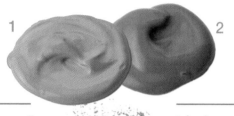

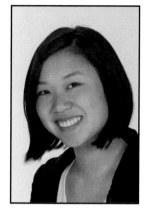

**elisha before**

## focal points

4 Use a **warm brown brow pencil** on brows. 5 Use a **taupe brown shadow** over lid. 6 I used a **shimmery green/gray color eye shadow** in layer 3 to create depth. 7 Apply **black eyeliner** on top lid adding extra on the top outer corners to create the illusion of lift. I also lined the lower lash line. Curl lashes and 8 apply **black mascara** to top and bottom lashes. 9 Add a few **short black individual lashes** on top outer corners.

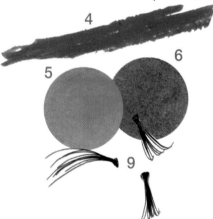

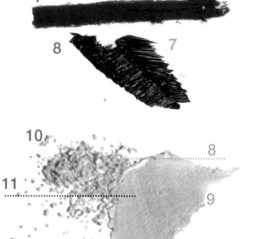

## focal points

4 Apply an **ashy brown brow cream** to accentuate brows. 5 Use **shimmery coral eye shadow** on eyelids creating a slightly winged effect at the outer corners of the eyes. This gives the eye a more modern edgy look. 6 Apply **black liner** on the top outer corners only. Curl lashes and 7 apply **black mascara** to top and bottom lashes.

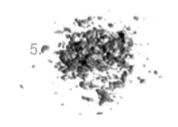

8 Apply **pink blush** to apples of cheeks. 9 Apply **cream highlighter** above apples and at temples.

For young girls I think less is more. 10 I applied a **shimmery pink lip gloss**. 11 Then I added more **clear lip gloss** for extra shine.

10 Apply **pink blush** to apples of cheeks. 11 Apply **cream highlighter** above apples and at temples.

12 Apply a **dark fleshtone liner** to create a balanced mouth, adding a few strokes to the center to create an even blend. 13 Apply a **berry cream lipstick** over entire mouth blending over the liner.

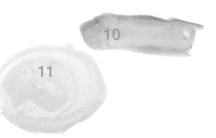

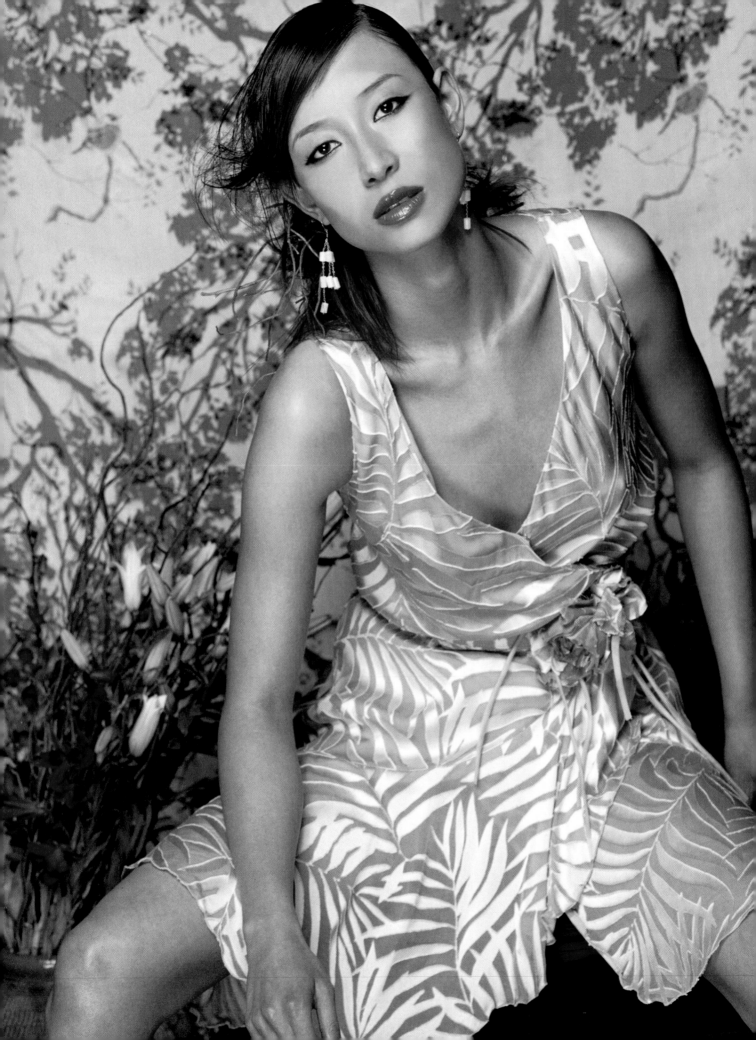

NIGHTTIME IS A great time to show off your best features. I love the nightlife, and how the mood in the city changes after the sun goes down. The dark always seems to bring out other sides of people's personalities. We can let go of our serious demeanors and do whatever we want—and look however we want. In the darker hours, you can have more fun with fashion and makeup—I love using great clothes as inspiration for makeup looks. Brighter shadows, lots of shimmer, and glossier lips are expected and even envied. That's what this chapter is all about; it's fashion-forward makeup; it's trendy, fun, and sexy. I believe that everyone has her own inner fashionista and nighttime is a perfect time to let her out. So play a little and have fun!

# night faces

# your special event

## Professional Facials

I was at a huge awards show one year and had to do a quick touch-up on a celebrity. She had gotten a facial two days prior to the event to look her best. She regularly received facials from the same place and used the same products, but for some reason this time she suffered a reaction and broke out in small bumps all over her face. Fortunately for her you couldn't see them unless you were a foot from her face. So I focused on just making her eyes and lips look great to take the focus off her skin. A good way to try to avoid any similar snafus before your next special occasion is to try to go for professional facials once a month in the time leading up to your event, making sure your last facial is about a month before the event itself.

If you happen to get a pimple (which I notice happens only before the most important events!), see your dermatologist for a cortisone shot. (This reduces the inflammation and makes it easier to cover up.) I also like to use products that contain benzoyl peroxide and sulfur to bring the pimple out from below the surface then away. (Sulfur brings the pimple to the surface and benzoyl peroxide dries it up. I usually sleep with it on.) Then make sure to cover up with the perfect concealer. If you feel that you absolutely have to pop a pimple (which I highly discourage), make sure your hands are squeaky-clean, clean the infected area with astringent and steam (get a bowl of hot water and put a towel over your head and allow the steam to open up your pores), then gently squeeze using finger cots (they're like finger gloves and are sold in pharmacies). I must warn you that popping pimples can infect nearby pores, leaving you with one old, inflamed pimple and some new ones as well. Take care of your skin before your big event, drink plenty of water, and relax.

## Waxing

Never get a facial wax on the day of your event. The skin on your face is covered in tiny facial hairs, and though you might not like the appearance of them, these hairs actually help foundation stay on and give the skin a softer finish. If you apply foundation to freshly waxed skin, you'll notice that the waxed area appears tough and shiny (kind of like the scalp that shows through on a bald head) instead of dewy and youthfully soft. To prevent this, make sure to get waxed no less than forty-eight hours before your event.

## Waterproof Yourself

Even if you hate waterproof mascara, it's better to be safe than sorry. For weddings especially, I only use waterproof eyeliner and mascara on everyone. I cry at every wedding even if I don't know the people.

**Cool Tip**

Dust a little shimmer powder over exposed collarbones and shoulders for an extra pop. Do this after getting dressed to avoid getting the powder all over your outfit.

## Touch-up Essentials

During your special event you are likely to take a very small bag with you that will only have enough room to hold your ID, a credit card, some cash, and a few makeup products. You should only need to carry three or four products with you if you've done the rest of your makeup correctly:

1. Pressed powder to avoid shine. Do not bring loose powder as it is more likely to create a mess and you probably don't have room to carry a powder brush as well.
2. Lipstick and lip gloss for quick touch-ups after eating.
3. Cotton swabs to clean up excess smudges and smears that may happen after laughing, crying, drinking, or hugging.

## Picture Perfect

There are always tons of pictures taken at special events. If you always look too white in photos it's because the flash reflects off makeup causing foundation to blow out to a lighter color. To avoid this, opt for a foundation that is half a shade darker than your regular foundation, and if your chest is exposed, make sure your face is the same color as your chest. If your chest is several shades darker, you can contour to match your chest without looking too dark (see page 61). Use sheer powders that don't contain too much shimmer as too much shimmer in photos can look greasy. Make sure to use a little extra powder in the T-zone area of your face, as this area tends to look very shiny in photos.

Shimmer will get blown out by flashes (similar to the sun glaring off the windshield of a car, but not as intense), so using shimmery shadows too close to the lash line may make your eyes appear smaller. Instead, use shimmers in layers 1 and 2 only and matte shadows in layers 3 and 4 (see pages 42 and 43).

## Teeth Whitening

I like to recommend beginning this process a month before your event. See your dentist before attempting any at-home treatments and make sure to use ADA-approved products. The strongest treatment is bleach (available only through dentists). Peroxide is available over-the-counter or from your dentist. These are actually great and whiten teeth significantly. They come in strips or moldable mouth guards. I prefer the guards because they form to your teeth and really whiten in-between teeth as well. Whitening toothpastes contain some abrasives that will remove surface stains. Many methods of teeth whitening can cause temporary sensitivity so don't do it too close to event time.

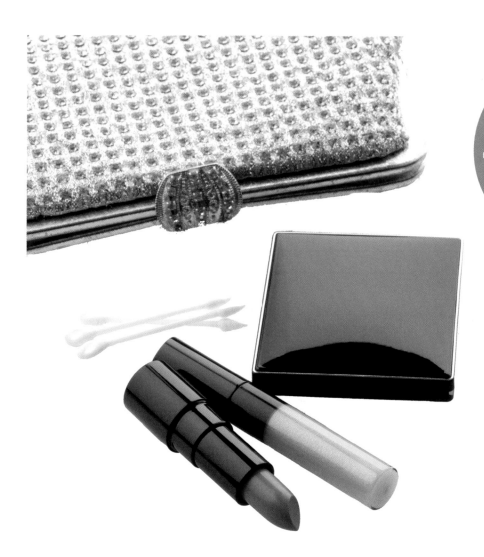

### Cool Tip
Brides, give your little purses to the person closest to you at your wedding—your mom, sister, or bridesmaid. You won't want to carry anything with you, and it'll give you a chance to reconnect with them.

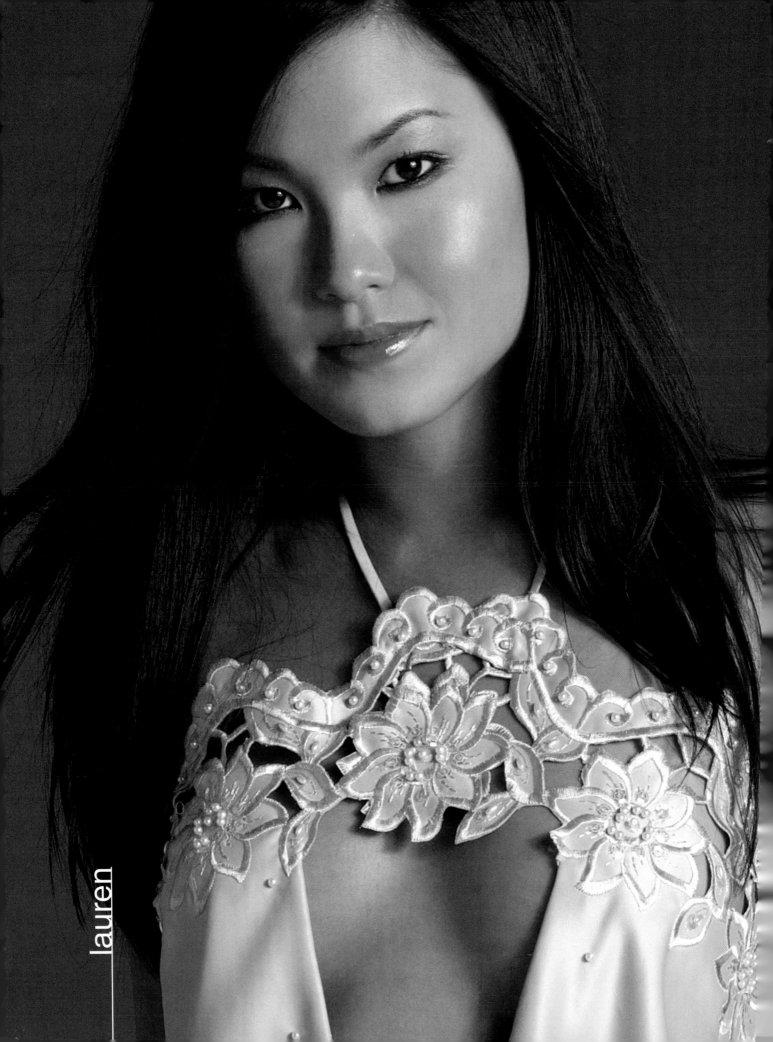

lauren

# saturday night

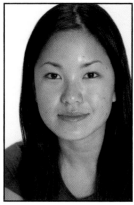

**lauren before**

1  Apply a highlight foundation to the center of the face.
2  Blend in a contour foundation to the outside of the face and eyelids.
3  Apply under-eye concealer where necessary.
4  Use a darker concealer for the skin.
5  Set with translucent yellow-based powder.
6  Apply ash brown brow cream to brows.
7  Use a teal-colored eyeliner around entire eye.
8  Apply black eyeliner.
9  Apply black mascara.
10  Apply apricot blush to apples of cheeks.
11  Apply cream highlighter above apples and at temples.
12  Apply neutral lip liner.
13  Apply warm apricot lip gloss.
14  Apply clear lip gloss.

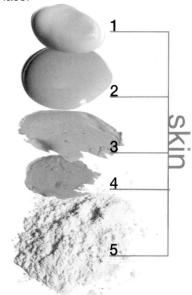

skin

## focal points

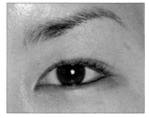

Create a natural contour to the lid using contour foundation on the eyelid (layer 2) set with powder. I used a **metallic teal-color eye pencil** around Lauren's entire eye. I blended above the crease to create an intense look and give the illusion of a larger lid. Apply **black eyeliner** along top and bottom lash line and inside the lower rim.

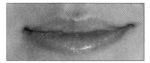

Lauren has pretty symmetrical lips. I softened the peaks with a **neutral lip liner** and added a **warm apricot lip gloss**, mixing it with **clear lip gloss** to create an even more glossy sheer look.

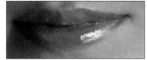

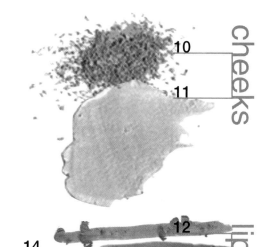

eyes

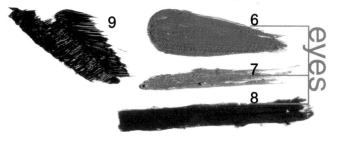

cheeks

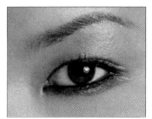

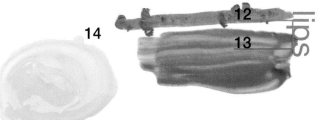

lips

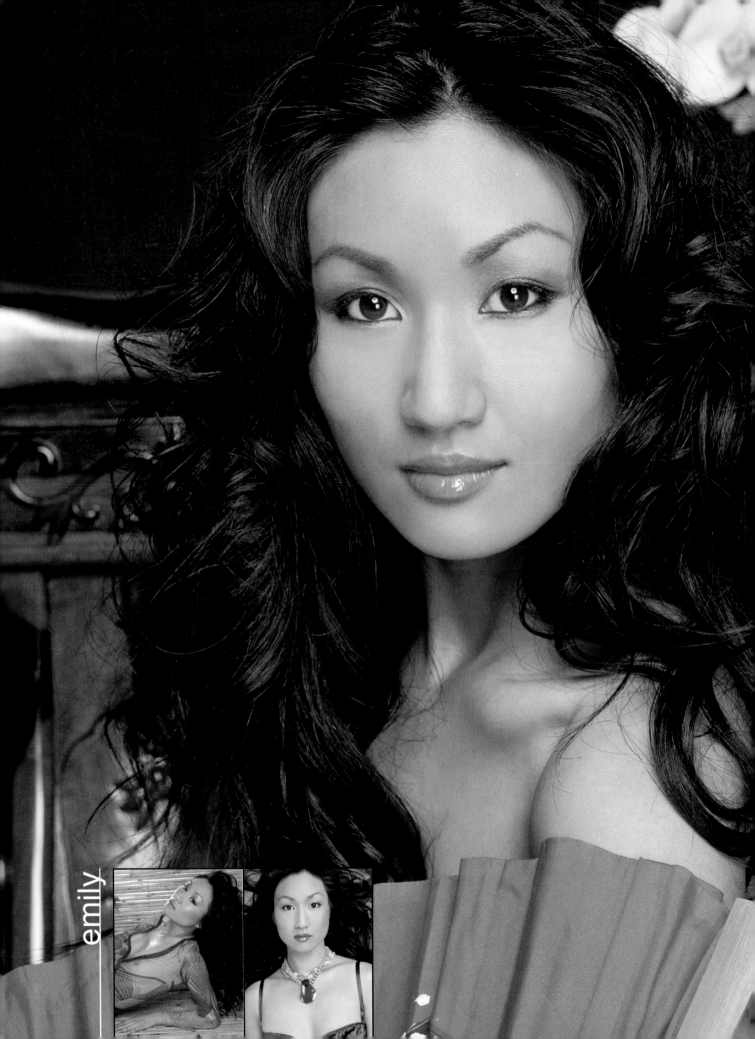

emily

# sultry

1 Apply a highlight foundation to the center of the face.
2 Blend in a contour foundation to the outside of the face.
3 Apply under-eye concealer where necessary.
4 Use a darker concealer for the skin.
5 Set with translucent yellow-based powder.
6 Apply warm brown brow pencil to brows.
7 Use a taupe brown shadow at base.
8 Use a lime green–colored eye shadow in layer 3.
9 Apply black eyeliner.
10 Apply black mascara.
11 Apply blush to apples of cheeks.
12 Apply cream highlighter above apples and at temples.
13 Apply neutral lip liner.
14 Apply sheer pink lip gloss.

## focal points

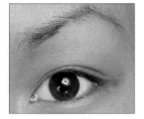 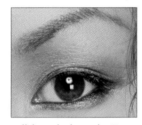

Use a **taupe brown shadow** over lid and along bottom lash line. I used a **shimmery lime green shadow** on layer 3 and just under the bottom lash line, slightly blending it with the existing **taupe shadow.** I applied **black liner** to the top lid and inside the lower rims, slightly smudging the liner along the lower lash line to create the illusion of a sultry larger eye. Curl lashes and finish with black mascara on top and bottom.

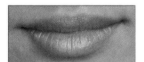 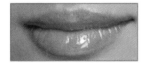

Emily has a slightly smaller upper lip, so I used **neutral lip liner** to gently draw above the natural lip line. I added a couple strokes of liner to the center of the mouth, then filled in the mouth with a **pink sheer lip gloss** blending over the lip liner.

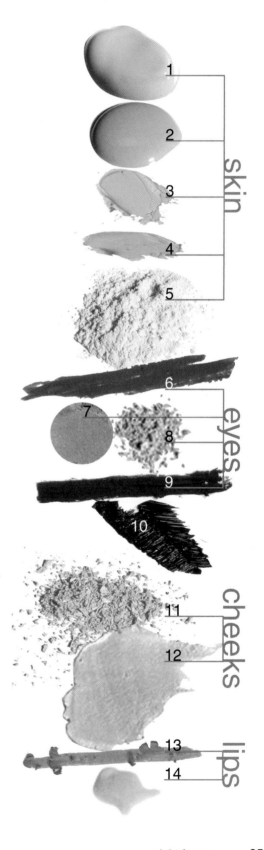

skin

eyes

cheeks

lips

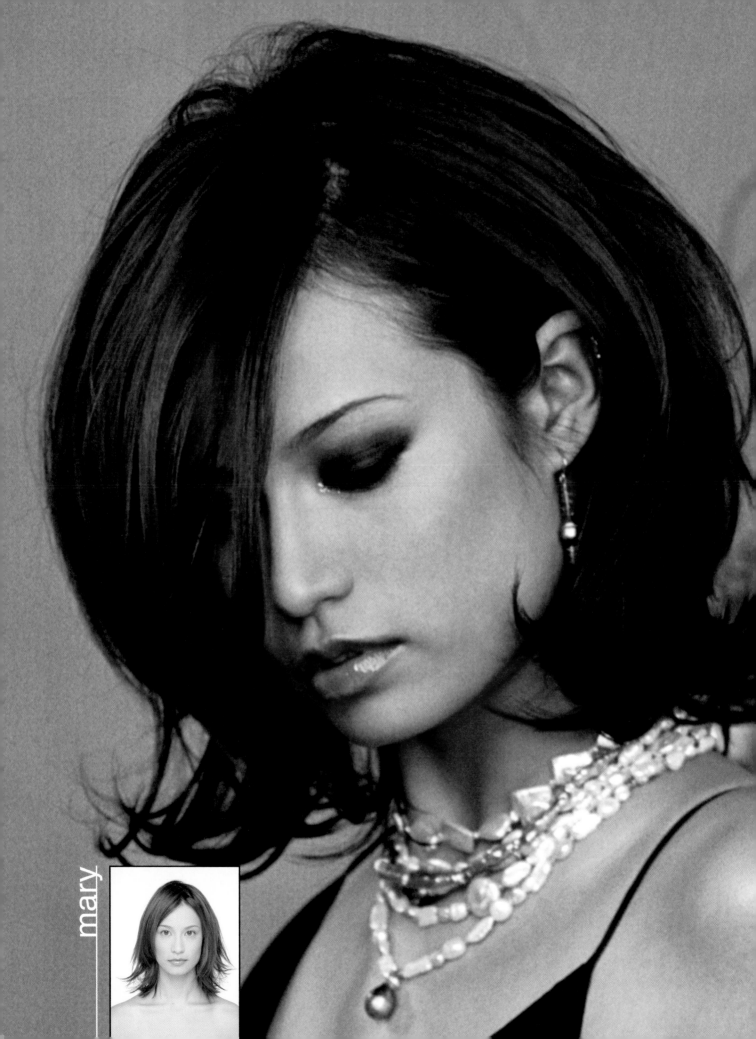

mary

# diamonds & pearls

1. Apply a highlight foundation to the center of the face.
2. Blend in a contour foundation to the outside of the face.
3. Apply under-eye concealer where necessary.
4. Set with translucent yellow-based loose powder.
5. Apply ash brown brow cream to brows.
6. Use a cool brown shadow at base.
7. Apply black eye shadow.
8. Apply black eyeliner.
9. Apply silver glitter.
10. Apply black mascara.
11. Apply a hint of rose blush to apples of cheeks.
12. Apply neutral lip liner.
13. Apply clear lip gloss.

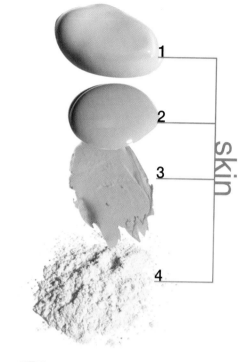

**skin**

## focal points

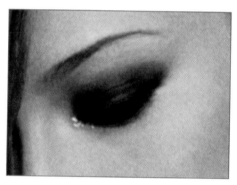

Use a **warm brown shadow** over lid (layer 2). I used a heavy application of **black eye shadow** in layer 3. (For a longer-lasting application, use black liner and set with black eye shadow.) I applied a thick line of **black liner** along top and bottom lash line and smudged it. Apply eyeliner inside lower rim.

Apply a hint of **silver glitter** to the inner corners of the eyes. Curl lashes and apply mascara to top and bottom lashes.

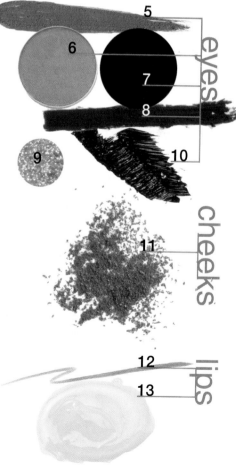

**eyes**

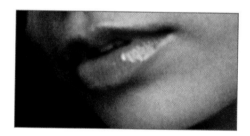

I lined Mary's entire lips with a **neutral lip liner** and blended in a **clear lip gloss**, allowing much of Mary's natural lip color to come through.

**cheeks**

**lips**

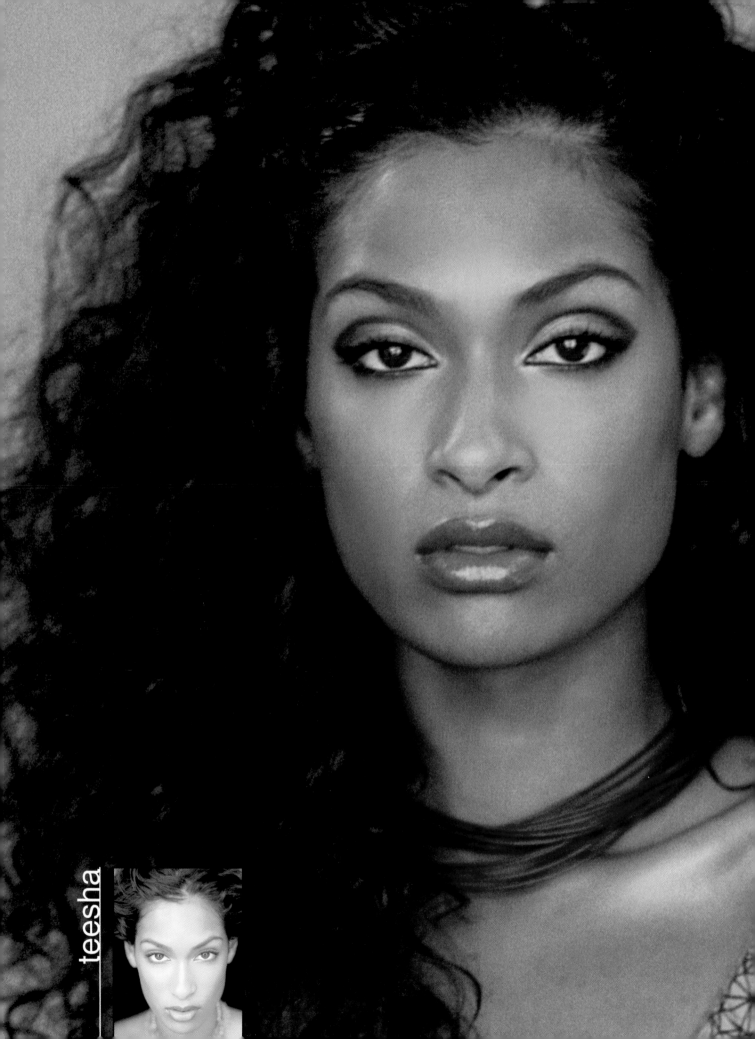

teesha

# eye candy

1. Apply a highlight foundation to the center of the face.
2. Blend in a contour foundation to the outside of the face.
3. Apply under-eye concealer where necessary.
4. Set with golden brown loose powder.
5. Apply ash brown brow cream to brows.
6. Apply brick cream shadow.
7. Apply gold shimmery eye shadow.
8. Apply black eyeliner.
9. Apply black mascara.
10. Apply apricot blush to apples of cheeks.
11. Apply cream highlighter above apples and at temples.
12. Apply warm brown lip liner.
13. Apply warm apricot gloss.

## focal points

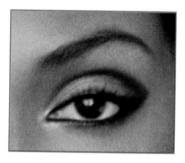

Use **brick-colored cream shadow** inside crease of upper lid and along the bottom lash line. I used **gold shimmery eye shadow** on the base of lid, brow bone, and inner corners of the eyes. Apply **black eyeliner** around entire eye including upper and lower rims of the eyes. Curl lashes and apply **black mascara** to top and bottom lashes.

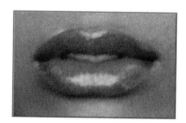

Apply a **warm brown lip liner** along natural lip line with a few strokes in the center. Blend in a **warm apricot lip gloss** over entire mouth.

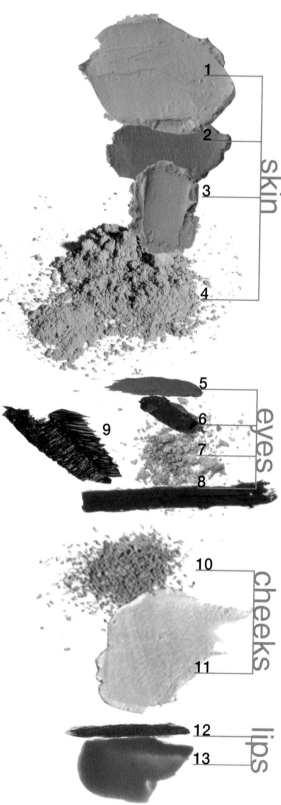

skin

eyes

cheeks

lips

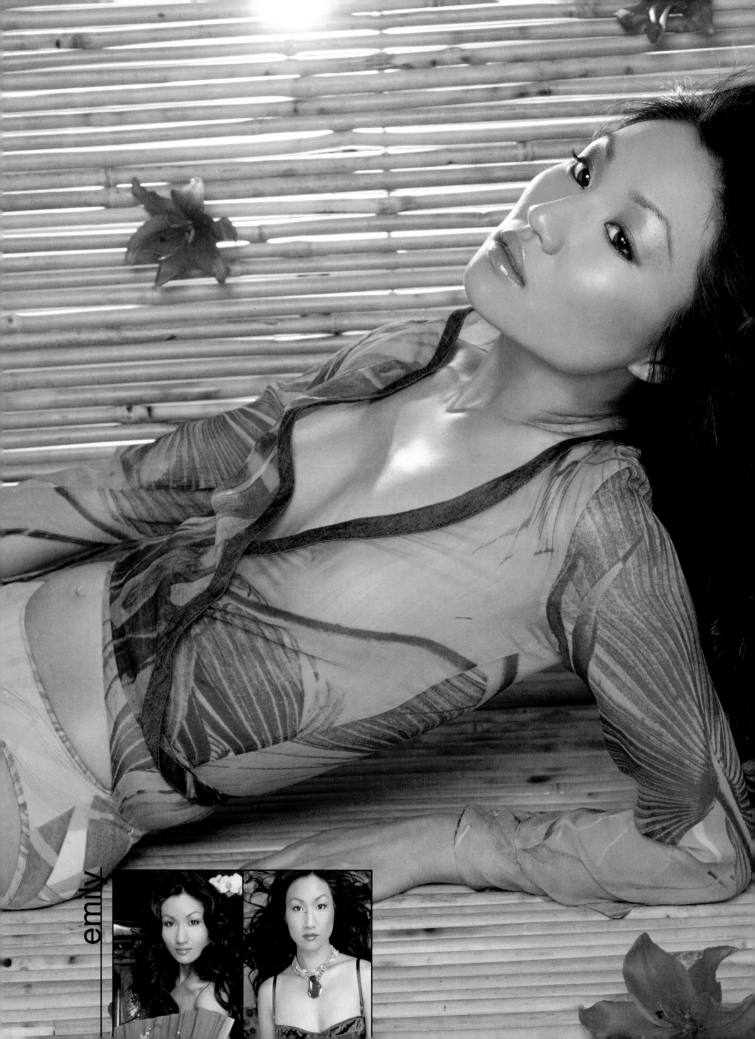

emily

# all that glitters

1  Apply a highlight foundation to the center of the face.
2  Blend in a contour foundation to the outside of the face.
3  Apply under-eye concealer where necessary.
4  Use a darker concealer for the skin.
5  Set with translucent yellow-based powder.
6  Apply warm brown brow pencil to brows.
7  Use a gold-colored shadow.
8  Use a bronze eye shadow.
9  Apply black eyeliner.
10  Apply black mascara.
11  Apply bronzer along cheekbones.
12  Apply cream highlighter above apples and at temples.
13  Apply beige shimmery lip gloss.

## focal points

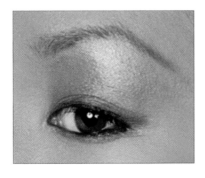

Use a **bronze shadow** over lid and along bottom lash line. I used a **shimmery gold eye shadow** on brow bone and inner corners of the eyes. I applied a **black liner** to top and bottom lash line, slightly smudging it to create a gentle smoke, then went over lash line again to intensify black line. Apply black liner to the lower rims. Curl lashes and apply **black mascara** to top and bottom lashes.

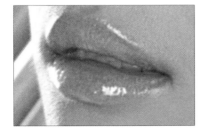

Apply **highlight foundation** over entire mouth to neutralize natural lip color. Apply a **beige shimmery** lip gloss over entire mouth.

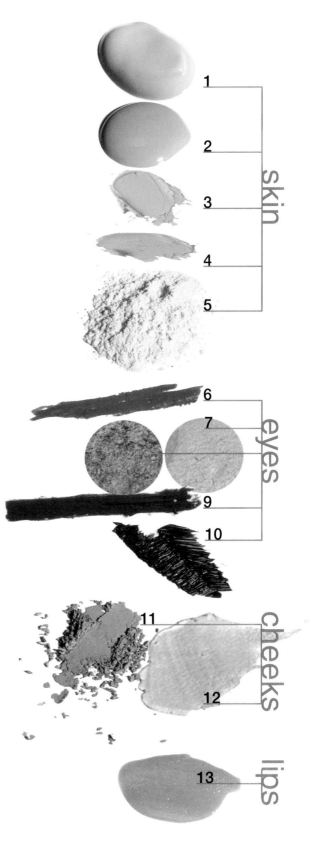

skin

1
2
3
4
5

eyes

6
7
9
10

cheeks

11
12

lips

13

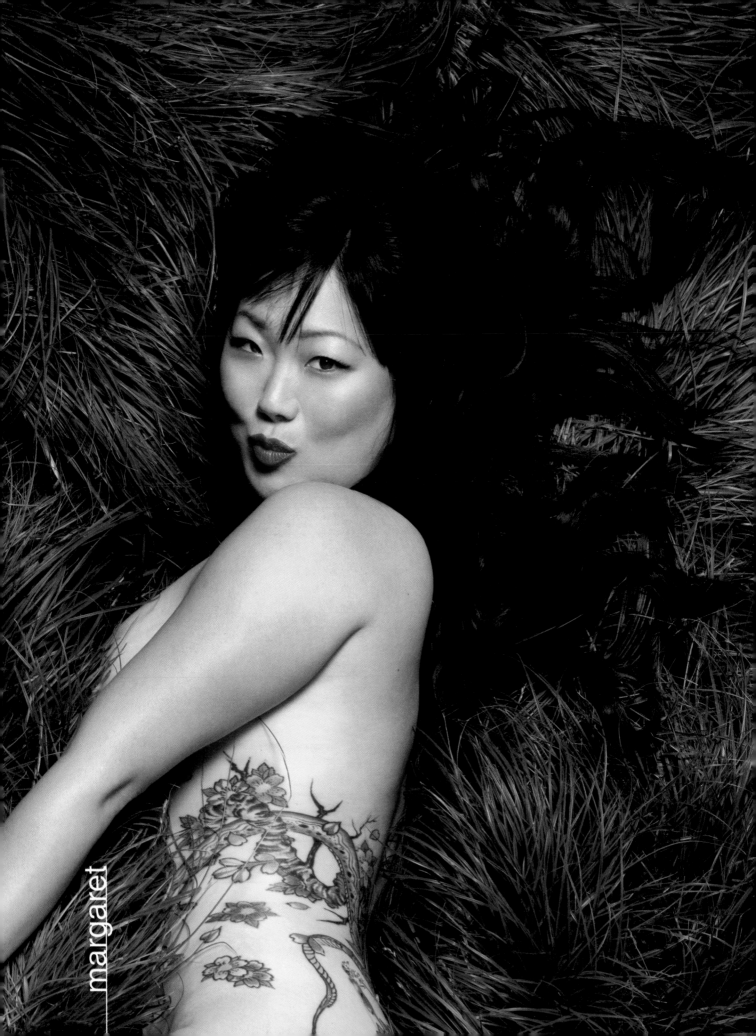

margaret

# stand-up glamour

*It was such a surreal moment doing Margaret Cho's makeup. I've watched her since I was a teenager—whether it was her stand-up, television show, or on the big screen. I am a huge fan. Margaret was always so funny to me because her stories were real. She understood what it was to be a Korean girl growing up in America, and she shared it with the world. Margaret broke the mold of Asian women being thought of as quiet and submissive. She is intelligent, voluptuous, funny, and strong. Beautiful.*

1  Apply a highlight foundation to the center of the face.
2  Blend in a contour foundation to the outside of the face.
3  Apply concealer where necessary.
4  Set with translucent powder.
5  Apply taupe brow pencil to brows.
6  Use a mauve eye shadow.
7  Use a pale shimmery shadow.
8  Apply black eyeliner.
9  Apply black mascara.
10  Apply three-quarter lashes.
11  Apply bright pink cream blush along cheekbones and temples, blend well.
12  Apply cream highlighter above apples and at temples.
13  Apply neutral lip liner.
14  Apply bright fuscia lipstick.

## focal points

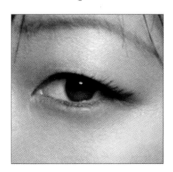

Apply a **taupe brow pencil** to create a soft arched brow. Apply a **pale shimmery shadow** over entire lid. Apply a **mauve eye shadow** in layer 3. Apply **black liner** along the lash line. Curl lashes and apply **black mascara** to top and bottom lashes. Finish with three-quarter lashes.

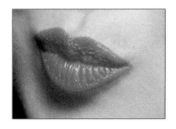

I slightly overdrew Margaret's mouth to create a sexy pout using a **neutral lip liner**. Then I covered the entire mouth with a **pink fuscia lipstick**.

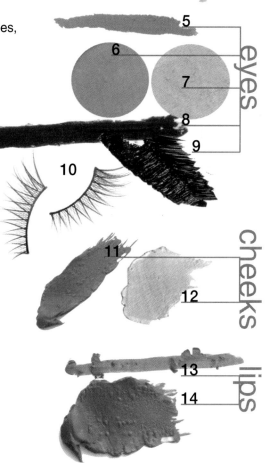

skin

eyes

cheeks

lips

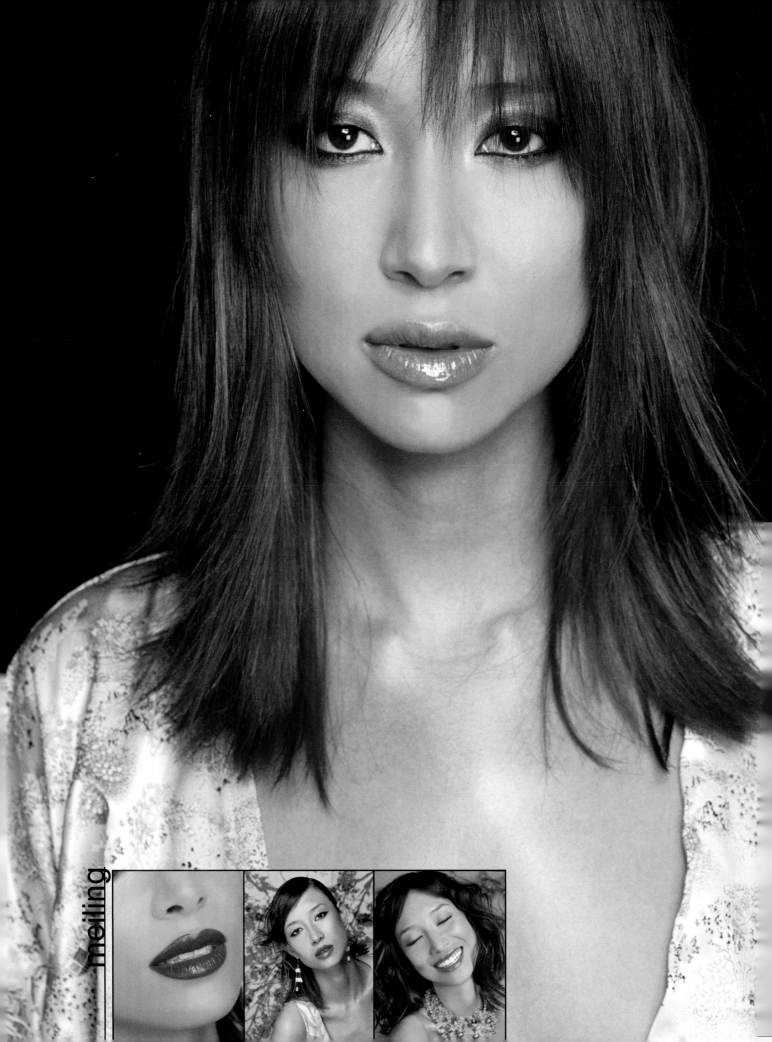

meiling

# kimono dragon

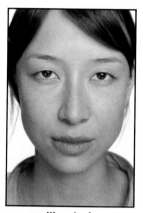

**meiling before**

1. Apply a highlight foundation to the center of the face.
2. Blend in a contour foundation to the outside of the face.
3. Apply under-eye concealer where necessary.
4. Set with translucent yellow-based loose powder.
5. Apply ash brown brow cream to brows.
6. Apply silver shadow at base.
7. Apply black shadow.
8. Apply black eyeliner.
9. Apply black mascara.
10. Apply pink blush to apples of cheeks.
11. Apply cream highlighter above apples and at temples.
12. Apply neutral lip liner.
13. Apply beige shimmery lip gloss.

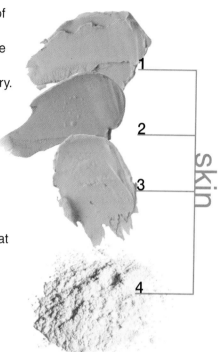

skin

## focal points

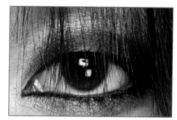

Use a **shimmery silver eye shadow** at base of the lid and along bottom lash line and inner corners of the eyes. Apply **black eye shadow** on layer 3 (this layering creates a smoky gray effect) and along bottom lash line. Apply **black eyeliner** along top and bottom lashes and inside lower rim. Curl lashes and apply mascara to top and bottom lashes.

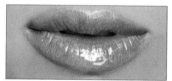

Use a **neutral lip liner** to slightly overdraw the top lip to create more symmetry. Apply **shimmery beige lip gloss** over entire mouth.

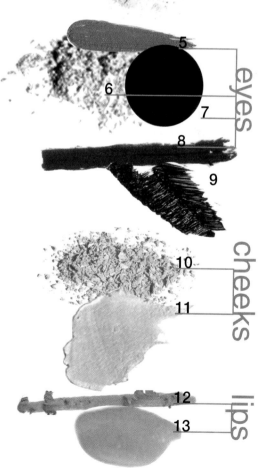

eyes

cheeks

lips

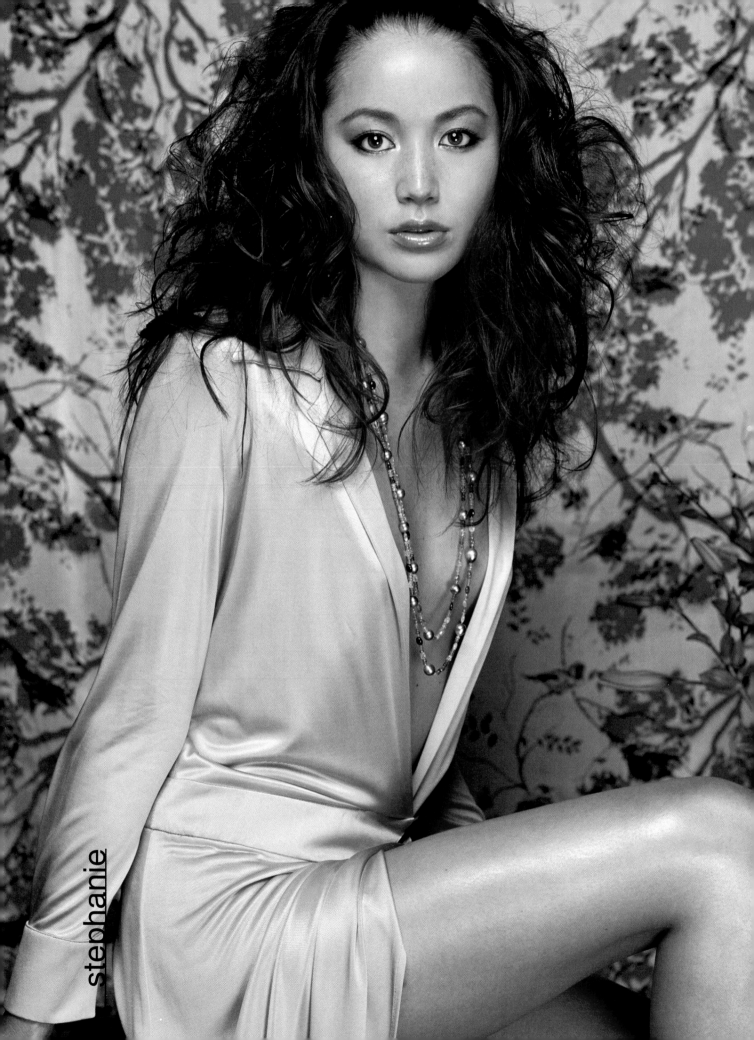

stephanie

# pretty in pinks

1 Apply a highlight foundation to the center of the face.
2 Blend in a contour foundation to the outside of the face.
3 Set with translucent yellow-based loose powder.
4 Apply ash brown brow cream to brows.
5 Use a warm pink eye shadow.
6 Use opal shadow at brow bone.
7 Apply white shimmery shadow in inner corners.
8 Apply black eyeliner.
9 Apply black mascara.
10 Apply warm salmon blush to apples of cheeks.
11 Apply neutral lip liner.
12 Apply pink opalescent lip gloss.
13 Apply clear gloss.

## focal points

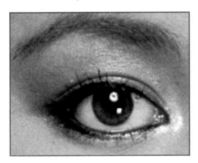

Use a **warm pink eye shadow** over base of eyelid and along lower lash line. Apply **opal shimmery shadow** along brow bone. Line top and bottom lash line with **black liner** and inside lower rim. Apply **white shimmery eye shadow** to the inner corners of the eyes. Curl lashes and apply **black mascara** to top and bottom lashes.

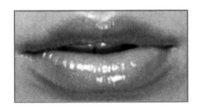

Line lips using a **neutral lip liner**. Apply an **opalescent pink lip gloss**. Finish with a **clear lip gloss** for intense shine.

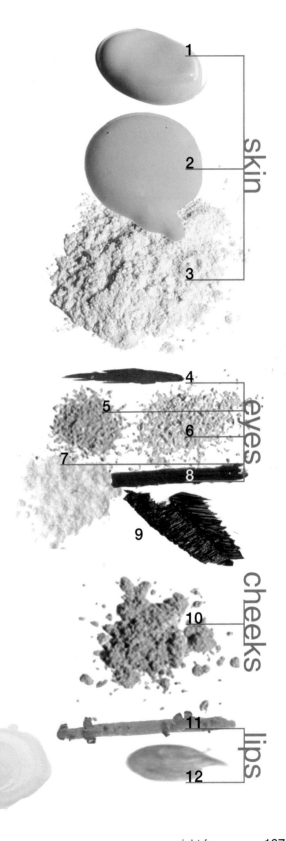

skin

eyes

cheeks

lips

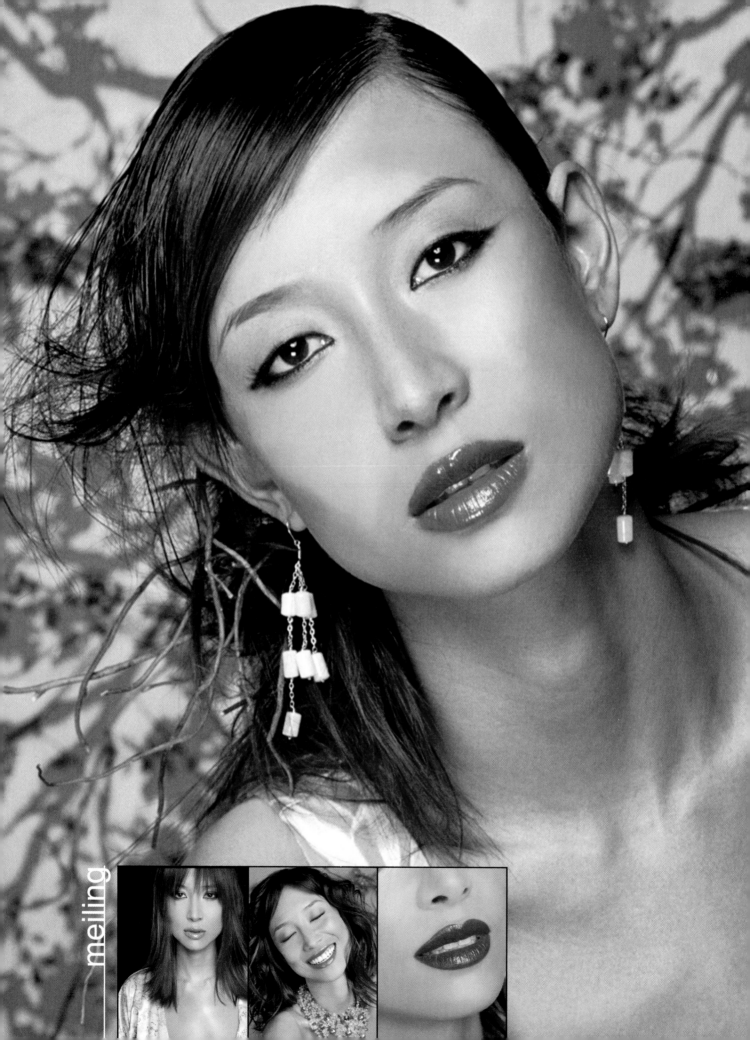

meiling

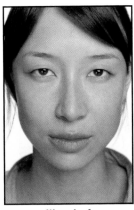

**meiling before**

1. Apply a highlight foundation to the center of the face.
2. Blend in a contour foundation to the outside of the face.
3. Apply under-eye concealer where necessary.
4. Set with translucent yellow-based powder.
5. Apply ash brown brow cream to brows.
6. Apply black eyeliner.
7. Apply shimmery white shadow on the inside corners of the eyes.
8. Apply black mascara.
9. Apply short individual lashes.
10. Apply warm salmon blush to apples of cheeks.
11. Apply cream highlighter above apples and at temples.
12. Apply neutral lip liner.
13. Apply warm plum lip gloss.

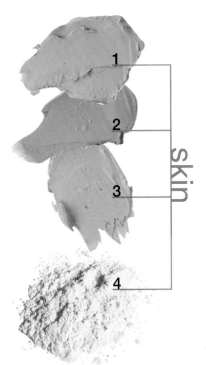

skin

## focal points

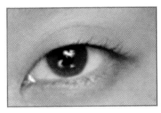 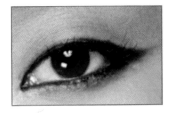

Apply **black eyeliner** around the entire eye and inside lower rims, winging out the outer corners. Apply **white shimmery shadow** to inner corners of the eyes. Curl lashes and apply **black mascara** to top and bottom lashes. Apply **short individual lashes** to outer corners of eyes.

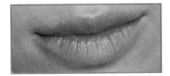 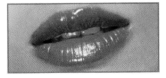

Line upper lip using a **neutral lip liner** to create a slightly rounded pouty effect. Apply **warm plum lip gloss** over entire mouth.

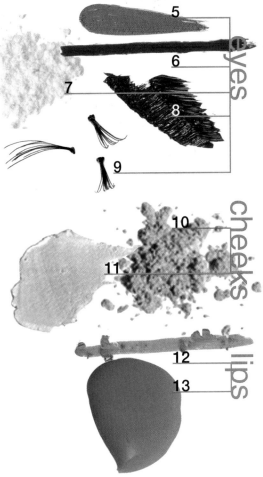

eyes

cheeks

lips

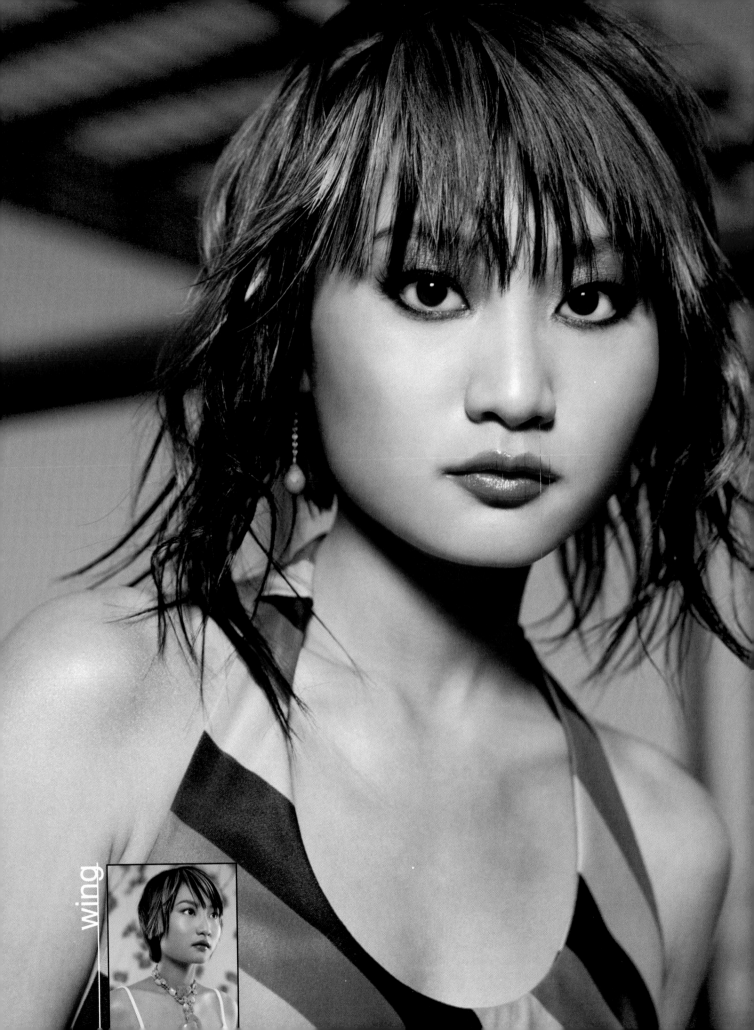

wing

# downtown girl

1 Apply opalescent highlighter to the entire face and neck.
2 Apply a highlight foundation to the center of the face.
3 Blend in a contour foundation to the outside of the face.
4 Apply under-eye concealer where necessary.
5 Use a darker concealer for the skin.
6 Set with translucent yellow-based loose powder.
7 Apply ash brown brow cream to brows.
8 Apply dark gold shadow at base.
9 Apply chestnut shadow.
10 Apply black eyeliner.
11 Apply black mascara.
12 Apply full strip false eyelashes.
13 Apply black liquid eyeliner.
14 Apply apricot blush to apples of cheeks.
15 Apply cream highlighter above apples and at temples.
16 Apply neutral lip liner.
17 Apply warm apricot lip gloss.

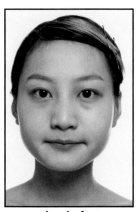

**wing before**

## focal points

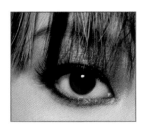

Apply **dark gold shadow** over entire lid leaving just the brow bone bare. Apply **chestnut brown shadow** at the base (layer 3). Apply a thick line of **black eyeliner** along the top and bottom lash line, slightly lifting up at the top outer corners. Apply **dark gold shadow** to the inner corners. Curl lashes and apply **black mascara** to top and bottom lashes. Apply **full strip false eyelashes**. Cover glue line after glue dries with **black liquid eyeliner.**

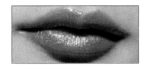

Wing has a smaller upper lip so I slightly overdrew the top using a **neutral lip liner**, lined the bottom lip along the natural lip line, added a few strokes of liner in the center, and blended in a **warm apricot lip gloss**.

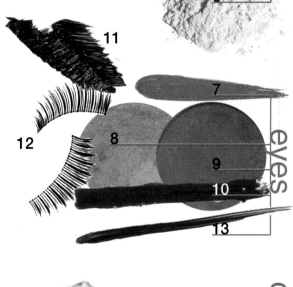

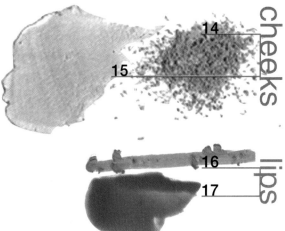

skin
eyes
cheeks
lips

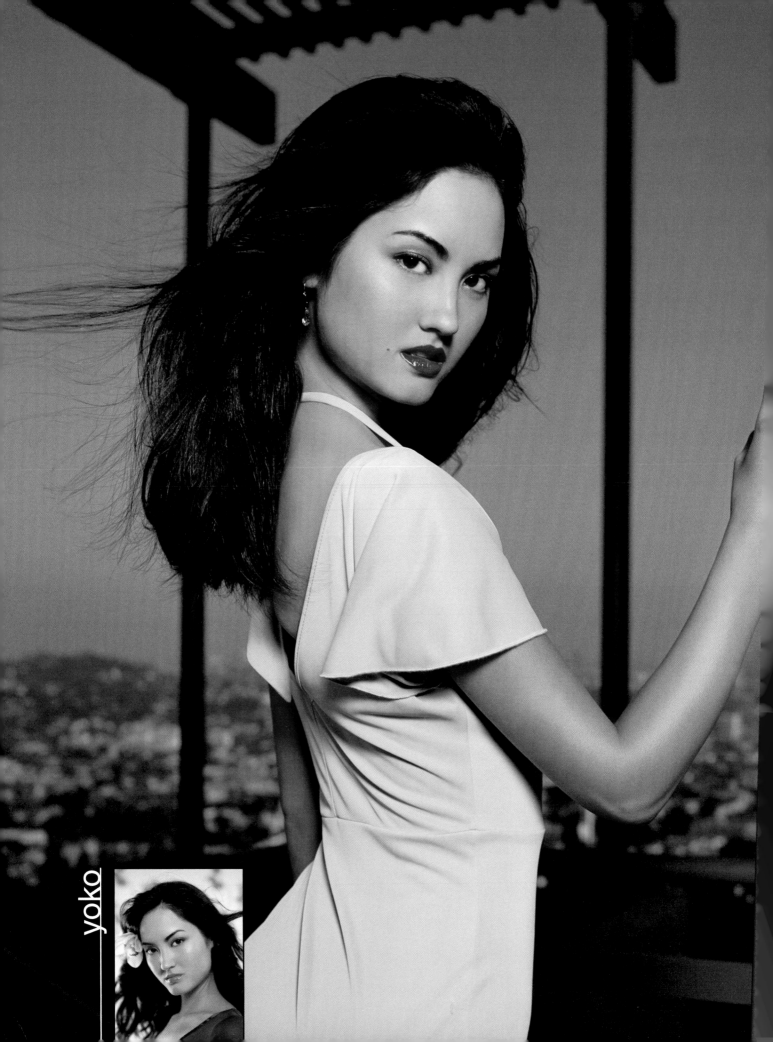

yoko

# rouged allure

1  Apply opalescent highlighter to the entire face and neck.
2  Apply a highlight foundation to the center of the face.
3  Blend in a contour foundation to the outside of the face.
4  Apply concealer where necessary.
5  Set with translucent yellow-based loose powder.
6  Apply dark brown brow powder to brows.
7  Use a dark gold cream eye shadow at base.
8  Apply black eyeliner.
9  Apply black mascara.
10  Apply pink blush to apples of cheeks.
11  Apply cream highlighter above apples and at temples.
12  Apply neutral lip liner.
13  Apply cherry red lipstick.
14  Apply clear lip gloss.

## focal points

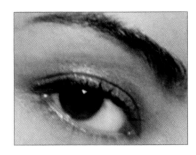

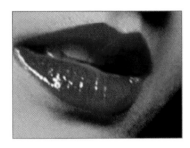

Use a **dark gold cream shadow** on base of lid (layer 2) and along the bottom end lash line. Apply **black liner** along top lash line beginning at the inner corners to the outer corner. Curl lashes and apply **black mascara** to top and bottom lashes.

I slightly overdrew Yoko's top lip using a **neutral lip liner**. Apply a **cherry red** lipstick over entire mouth. Add just a hint of **clear lip gloss**.

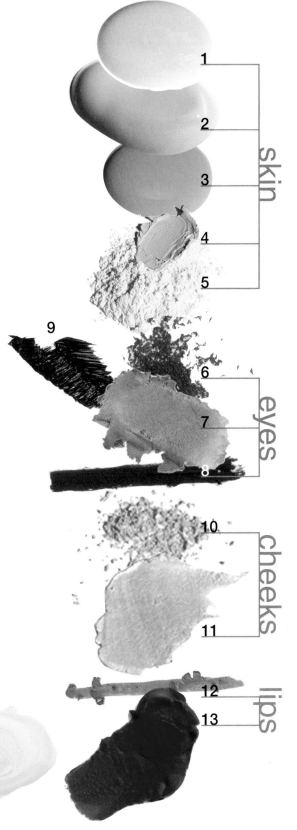

skin

1
2
3
4
5

9

6
7
8

eyes

10
11

cheeks

12
13

lips

14

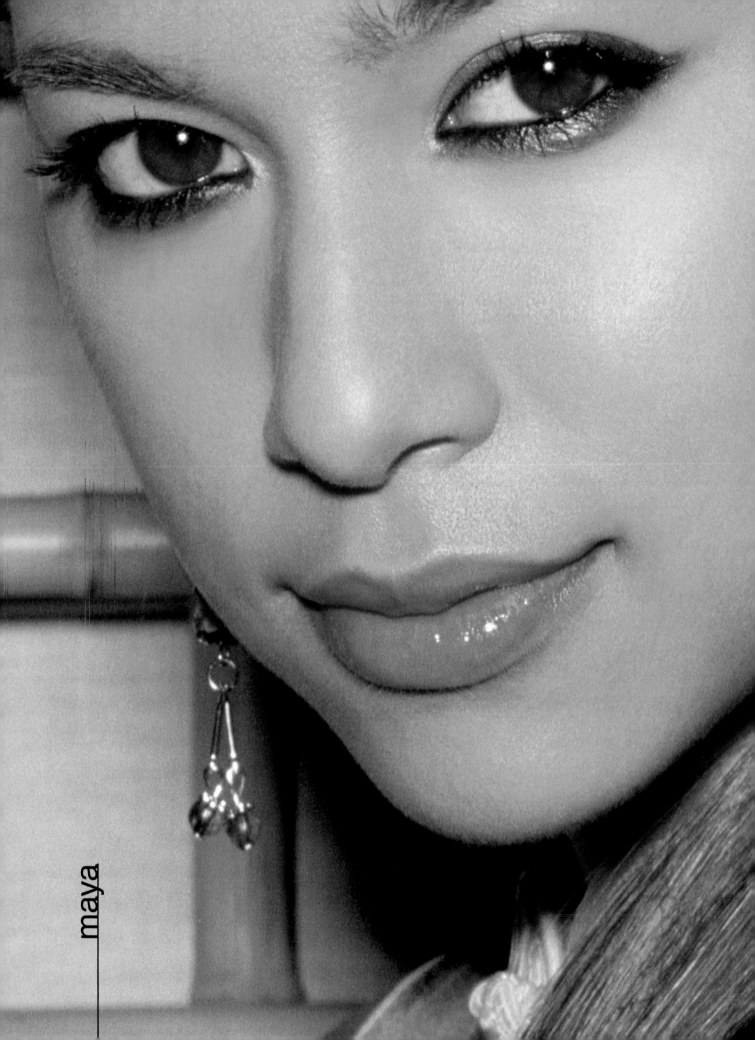

maya

# smoldering

1. Apply a highlight fluid foundation to the center of the face.
2. Blend in a contour fluid foundation to the outside of the face.
3. Apply under-eye cake concealer.
4. Set with translucent powder.
5. Apply ash brown brow cream to brows.
6. Use a taupe shimmery liner all around the eye.
7. Use a black pencil eyeliner to create a smoky eye.
8. Apply an off-white shimmer liner to the inner corner of the eye.
9. Apply black mascara to top and lower lashes.
10. Apply an apricot blush to apples of cheeks.
11. Apply cream highlighter above apples and at temples.
12. Use a warm lip liner to add definition to mouth.
13. Finish with a warm peach lip gloss.

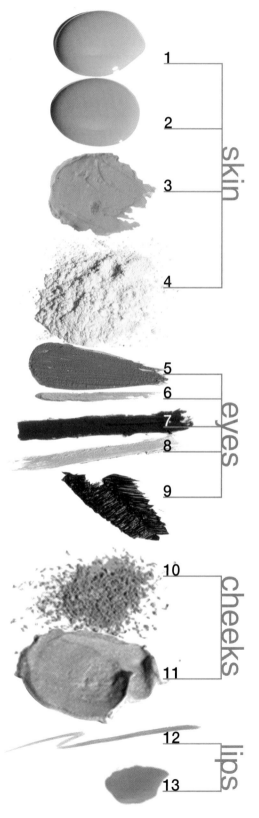

1
2
3 skin
4

5
6
7 eyes
8
9

10
11 cheeks

12
13 lips

## focal points

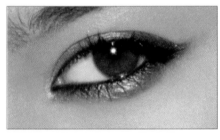

Use a **taupe shimmery eyeliner** all around the eye (layer 3). (You can also use most other eyeliner colors to create a clean smoky look.) Gently create a smoky eye by applying **black eyeliner** close to the upper and lower lash line. Smudge eyeliner almost completely into layer 3 using an **eyeliner smudge brush**. Add definition to the eye by applying a second coat of eyeliner inside the upper and lower rims. Apply an off-white shimmery liner to the inner corner of the eyes. Finish the look with mascara on upper and lower eyelashes.

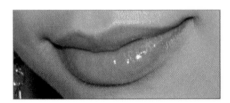

Apply a warm **neutral lip liner** to add definition to the mouth. Finish with a **warm peach lip gloss**.

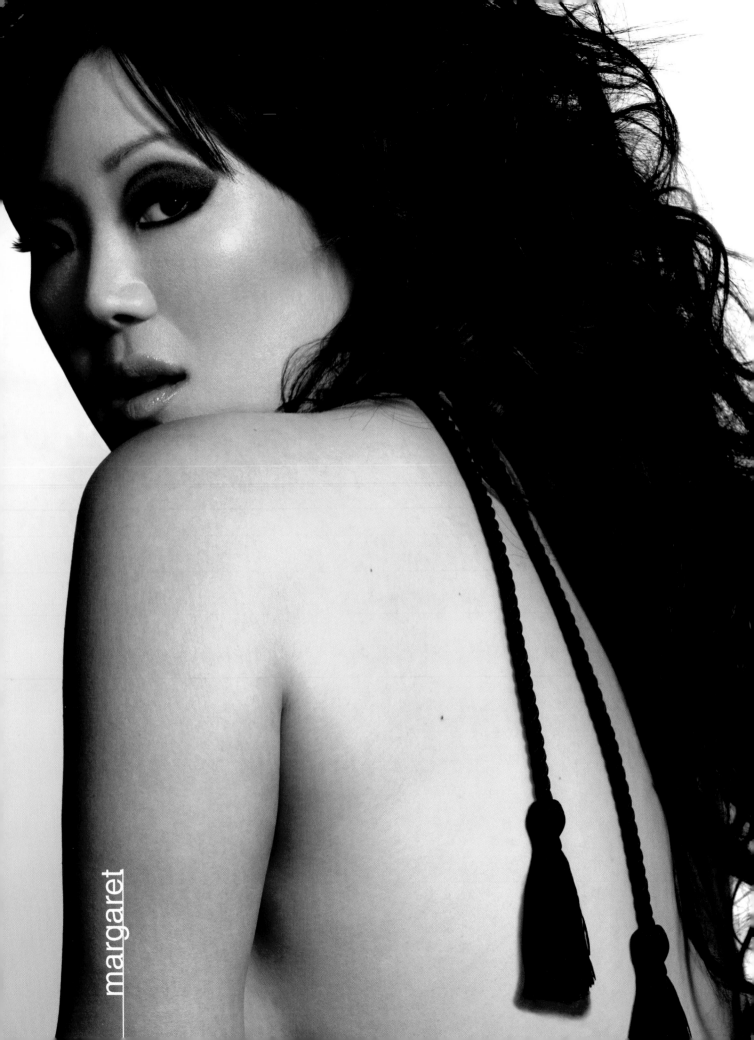

margaret

# extreme

1 Apply a highlight fluid foundation to the center of the face.
2 Blend in a contour fluid foundation to the outside of the face.
3 Apply under-eye cake concealer.
4 Set with translucent powder.
5 Apply ash brown brow cream to brows.
6 Use several layers of black eye shadow.
7 Apply purple cream shadow.
8 Use a black pencil eyeliner pencil to define a smoky eye.
9 Apply black mascara to top and lower lashes.
10 Apply full set of false eyelashes.
11 Apply bronzer along the cheekbone.
12 Apply cream highlighter above apples and at temples.
13 Use a neutral lip liner to add definition to mouth.
14 Finish with a clear lip gloss.

## focal points

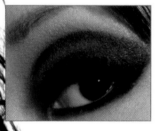

Apply an **ashy brown eyebrow pencil**. Apply several layers of **black eye shadow**, going into layers 2 and 3 as well as underneath the eye. Apply **purple cream eye shadow** just slightly along the underside rim of layer 2 for added color. Apply **black eyeliner** inside the lower rim and extend out to create a winged eye. Curl lashes and apply **black mascara** to top and bottom lashes. Apply a **full strip of false eyelashes** to the top lashes.

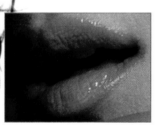

Apply a warm **neutral lip liner** to add definition to the mouth and fill in to create a neutral lip. Finish with **clear lip gloss**.

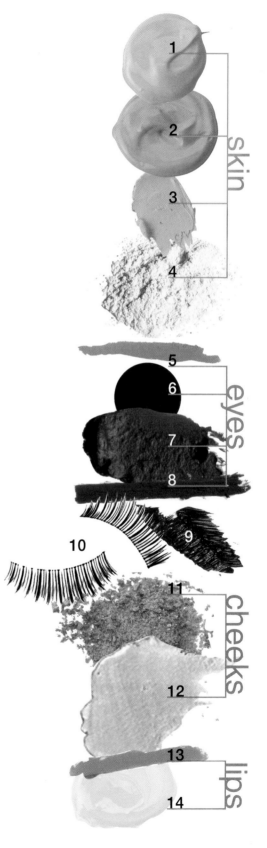

skin

1
2
3
4

eyes

5
6
7
8

10
9

cheeks

11
12

lips

13
14

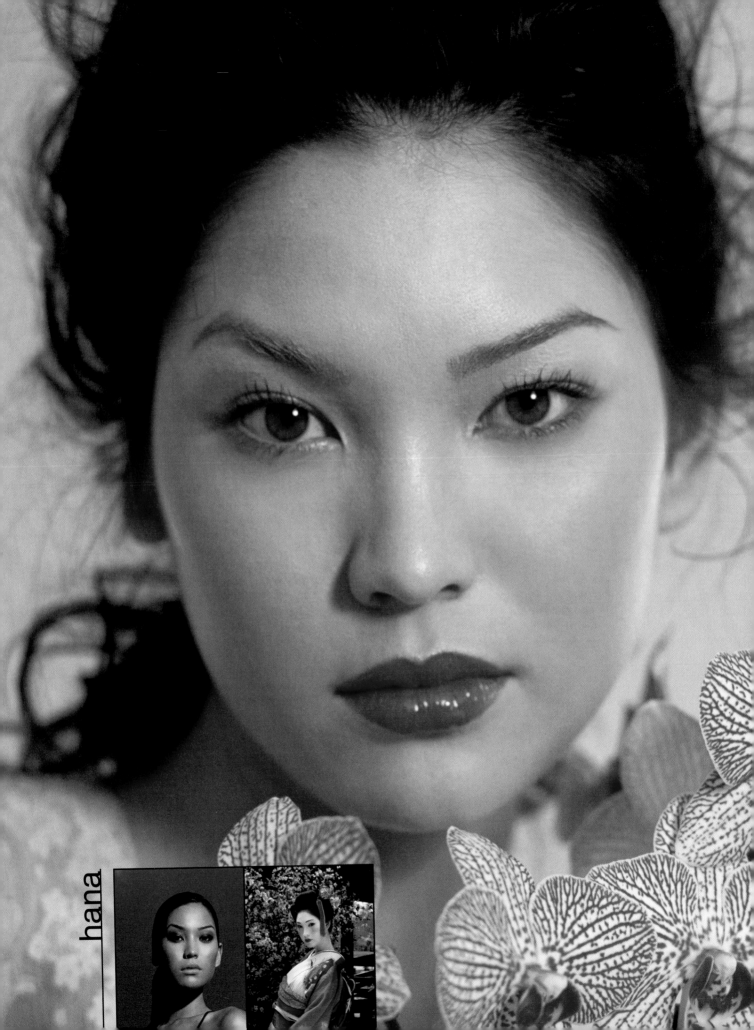

hana

1 Apply a highlight foundation to the center of the face.
2 Blend in a contour foundation to the outside of the face.
3 Apply under-eye concealer where necessary.
4 Set with translucent yellow-based powder.
5 Apply ash brown brow cream to brows.
6 Apply gold shimmery shadow on top of brows to lighten.
7 Apply yellow cream shadow.
8 Apply green eyeliner.
9 Apply black liquid eyeliner.
10 Apply black mascara.
11 Apply warm pink blush to apples of cheeks.
12 Apply fuscia lip liner.
13 Apply fuscia lipstick.

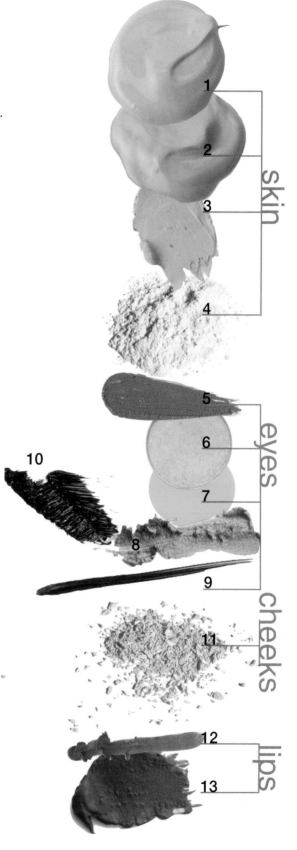

skin

eyes

cheeks

lips

## focal points

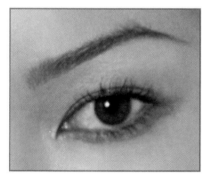

Use **ash brown cream shadow** to create a perfectly angled brow. Apply **pale gold shadow** on top of brows to lighten them. Apply **yellow cream eye shadow** over entire lid. Apply **green liner** along lower lash line. Apply a thin line of **black liquid liner** along the top lash line. Curl lashes and apply **black mascara** to top and bottom lashes.

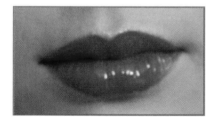

Line entire mouth using a **fuscia lip liner**. Blend a **creamy fuscia lipstick** over entire mouth.

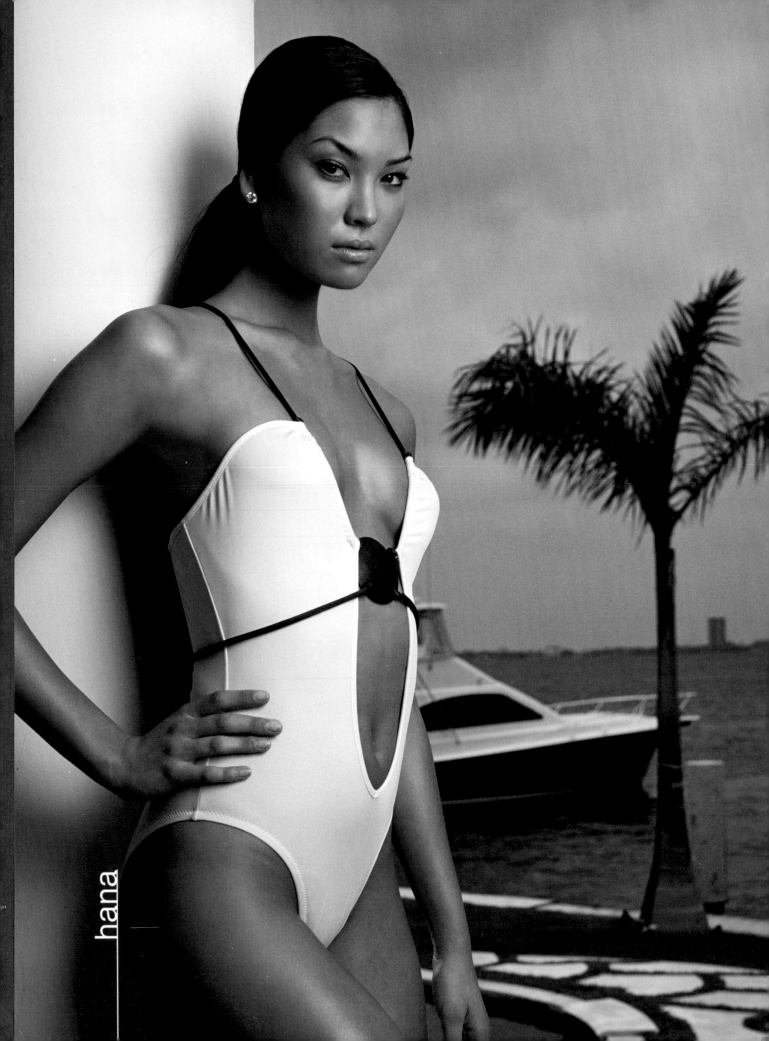

hana

*I love this very sexy city. Almost every woman in this town is a walking goddess. The look here is very high fashion, with dark skin and glossy makeup. Looking sexy while wearing minimal makeup can be a bit tricky, but the women here make it work. When I was there I didn't bother wearing any powder or foundation. I focused on gel bronzer and contouring with concealer to get intense color and a little lasting coverage. The makeup focus in Miami is on skin and sexy eyes. If you don't want to look like a tourist, even the palest skin needs a little spray tan.*

1  Apply a highlight foundation to the center of the face.
2  Blend in a contour foundation to the outside of the face.
3  Apply under-eye concealer where necessary.
4  Set with shimmery golden loose powder (optional).
5  Apply brown brow pencil to brows.
6  Use a copper cream shadow at base.
7  Use a gold cream eye shadow at the brow bone.
8  Apply black eyeliner.
9  Apply beige pink eyeliner.
10  Apply black mascara.
11  Short individual black eyelashes.
12  Apply cream bronzer along the cheekbone.
13  Apply cream highlighter above apples and at temples.
14  Apply neutral lip liner.
15  Apply fleshtone lipstick.

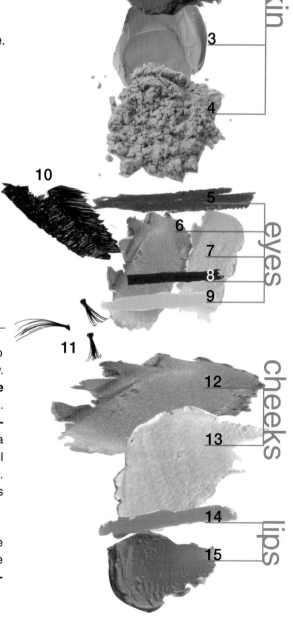

skin

eyes

cheeks

lips

## focal points

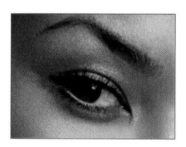

Use a **brown brow pencil** to accentuate the arch of the brow. Apply a **copper cream eye shadow** at the base of the lid. Apply a **gold cream eye shadow** at the brow bone. Apply a thin line of **black eyeliner** pencil to the top and bottom lash line.

Use a **beige pink liner** and line the inside lower rim. Curl lashes and apply **black mascara** to the top and bottom lashes.

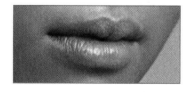

Apply **neutral lip liner** to define the natural lip line and fill in the entire mouth. Finish with **fleshtone lip color**.

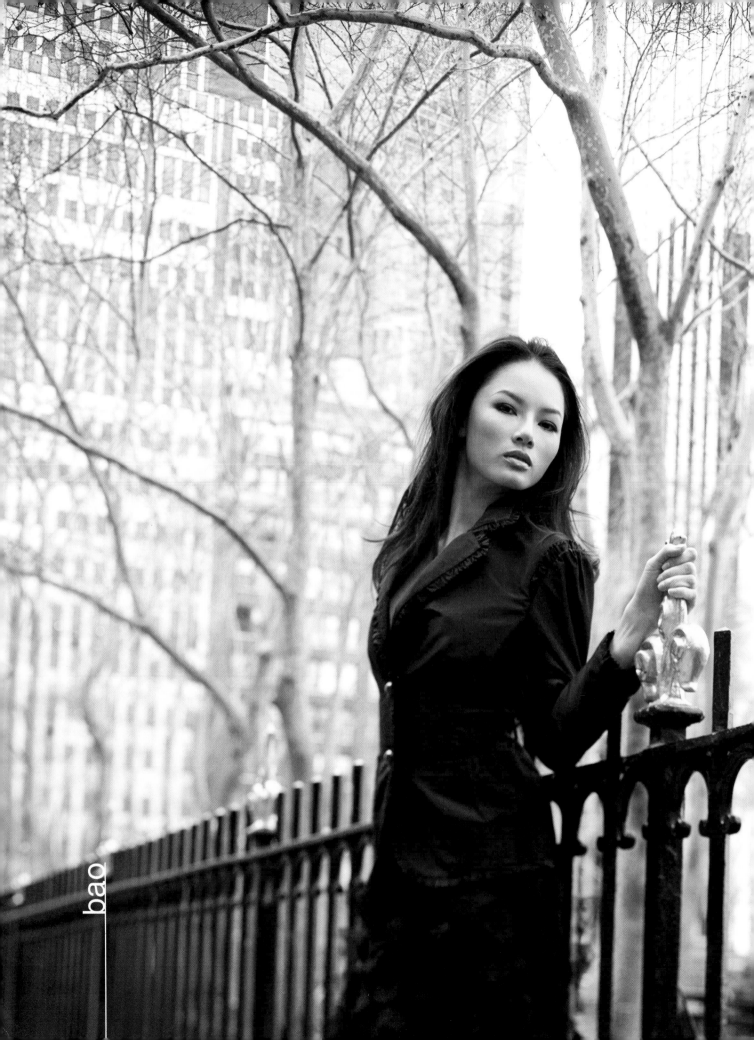

*Women in this city look sophisticated in a very understated way. Even glamorous styles are still very elegant. Makeup is minimal, sexy is replaced by sultry and classic. Look for deep red or neutral lip colors and avoid bright colors like fuscia and overglossed lips. False eyelashes should look natural. The look is fresh not flashy, polished without looking like you tried.*

1. Apply a cream foundation all over the face.
2. Blend in a contour foundation to the hairline. Contour the nose and cheekbones.
3. Apply under-eye concealer to under-eye circles and to lips to neutralize dark lips.
4. Set with translucent powder.
5. Apply ash brown brow pencil (5a) to the start of brows and dark ash (5b) to the ends.
6. Use a neutral brown shadow at base (I used the same color as bronzer).
7. Use a slightly darker brown in layer 3.
8. Apply chocolate brown eyeliner.
9. Apply beige eyeliner to inner rims to neutralize red eyes.
10. Curl lashes and apply black mascara.
11. Apply bronzer along the cheekbone.
12. Apply cream highlighter above apples and at temples.
13. Apply lip balm.
14. Use a warm neutral lip liner for definition.
15. Apply warm pink cream lipstick.

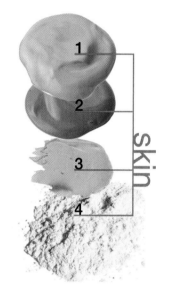

skin

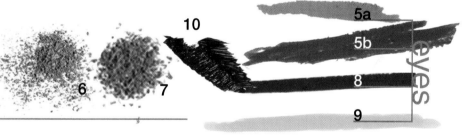

eyes

## focal points

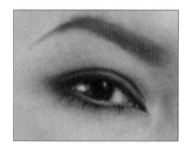

Use a **neutral brown shadow** to cover base of lid (layer 2). Use a slightly darker warm brown shadow for more depth (layer 3). Use a **chocolate brown pencil eyeliner** around the entire eye. Apply a **beige eyeliner** inside the lower rim. Curl lashes and apply **black mascara** to top and bottom lashes.

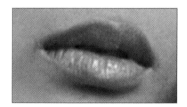

Apply **lip balm** to soften lips. Use a **warm neutral lip liner** to give definition to lips. Apply a warm **pale pink cream lipstick** to create a sophisticated look that's perfect for New York.

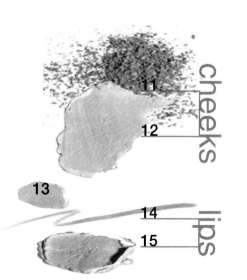

cheeks

lips

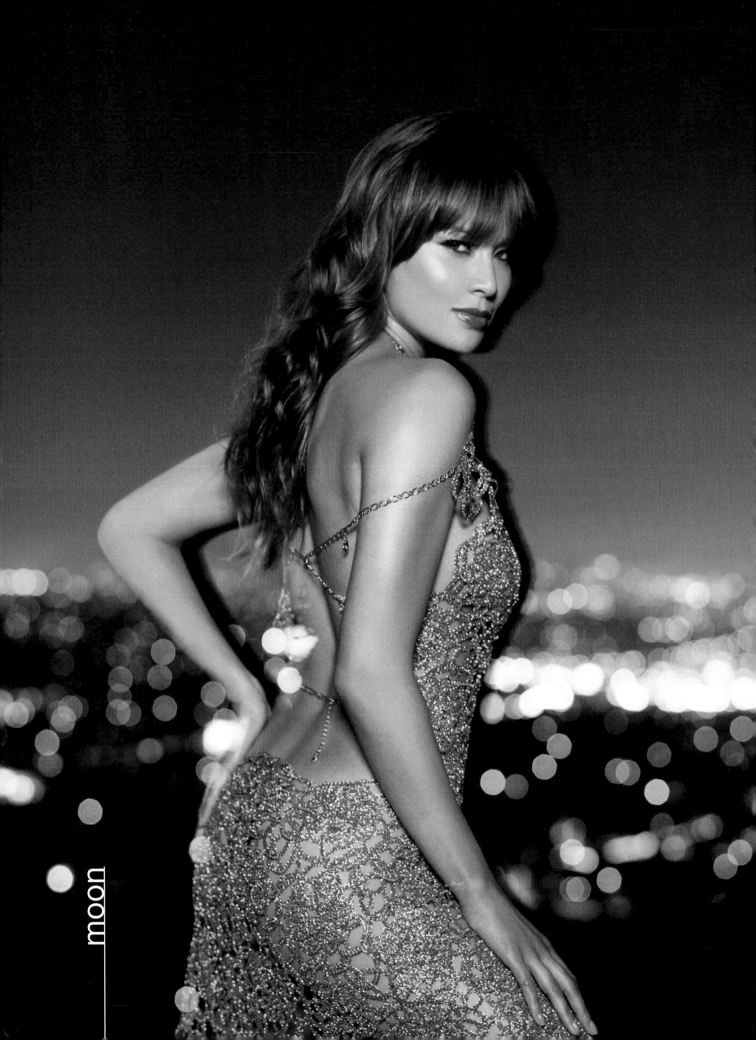

moon

*L.A. is the only city where you can go to an incredibly expensive restaurant and see people eating in sweats, and the next night head out to a major Hollywood event highlighted by magnificent gowns and high glamour. However, don't misunderstand me; even in sweats and their hair in a ponytail the women here will go all-out on their makeup. Too much is never enough when you're in the land of the rich and famous! I prefer smoky eyes in brown and blacks, paired with extremely glossy lips in nude colors, or clean sexy eyes with a dark lipstick in berries, bricks, and reds.*

1 Apply a highlight foundation to the center of the face.
2 Blend in a contour foundation to the outside of the face.
3 Apply under-eye concealer where necessary.
4 Use a darker concealer for the skin.
5 Set with translucent powder.
6 Apply strawberry brown brow cream to brows.
7 Apply black eyeliner.
8 Apply black mascara.
9 Apply individual lashes.
10 Apply bronzer along the cheekbone.
11 Apply cream highlighter above apples and at temples.
12 Apply dark berry cream lipstick.

## focal points

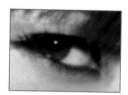

Use a **black eyeliner** around the entire eye. Curl lashes and apply **black mascara**. Apply **short black individual lashes** on the ends of the top outer corners of the eyes.

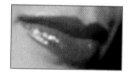

Moon has great symmetrical lips naturally. So I simply applied a **dark berry creamy lipstick** using a **lip brush** to achieve a perfect application.

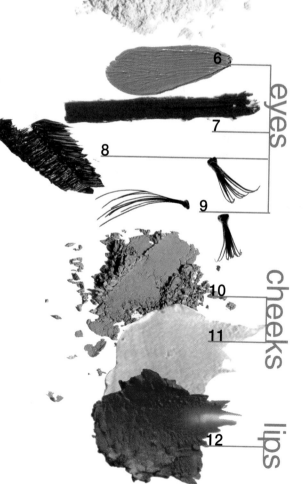

skin

eyes

cheeks

lips

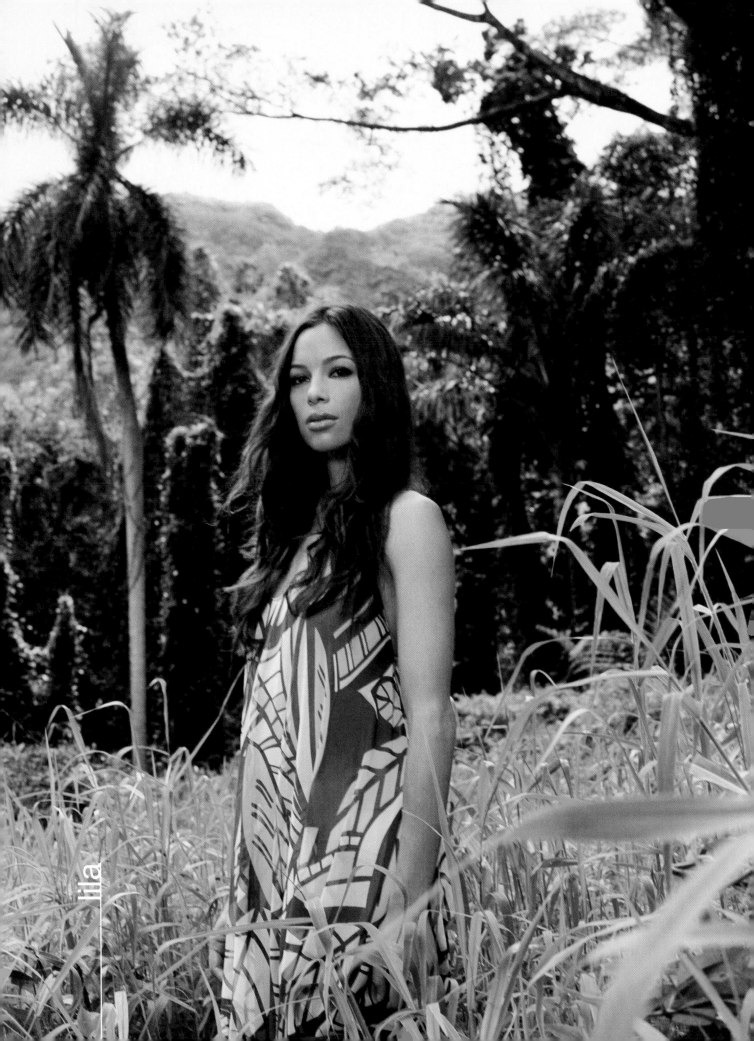

lila

*If I had to choose one word to describe Honolulu it would be tropical, lush, gorgeous—okay, that's three words. The first time I visited Hawaii for a job, we had problems with the weather. We would chase the sun while the rain chased us. Because of all the rain, I thought I would be fine with a low SPF sunscreen, but I still got severely burned. A sunscreen with a SPF 30 or higher is the way to go here. You're in a land that relishes long days at the beach and festive, informal luaus, so makeup should be kept very minimal: A little liner and mascara (waterproof, of course) and even a bit of shadow and some tinted lip balm and you're done. If you're going to wear blush, try cream or gel and keep it light.*

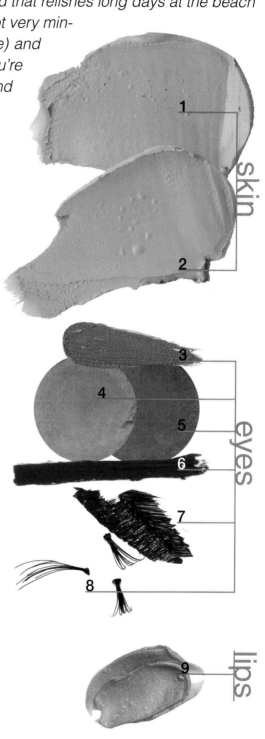

1  Apply a highlight foundation to the center of the face.
2  Blend in a contour foundation to the outside of the face.
3  Apply ash brown brow cream to brows.
4  Use taupe brown shadow at base.
5  Use chestnut brown shadow at base.
6  Apply black eyeliner.
7  Apply black mascara.
8  Apply short black individual lashes.
9  Apply warm pink lip gloss.

## focal points

Use a **taupe brown shadow** over base of the lid. Apply **chestnut brown shadow** to layer 3 and along the bottom lash line. Apply **black eyeliner** around the entire eye and inside the lower rim. Curl lashes and apply **black waterproof mascara**. I applied **individual lashes** along the top lash line (hey, it's a photo shoot).

Apply a **shimmery sheer copper lip gloss** over entire mouth.

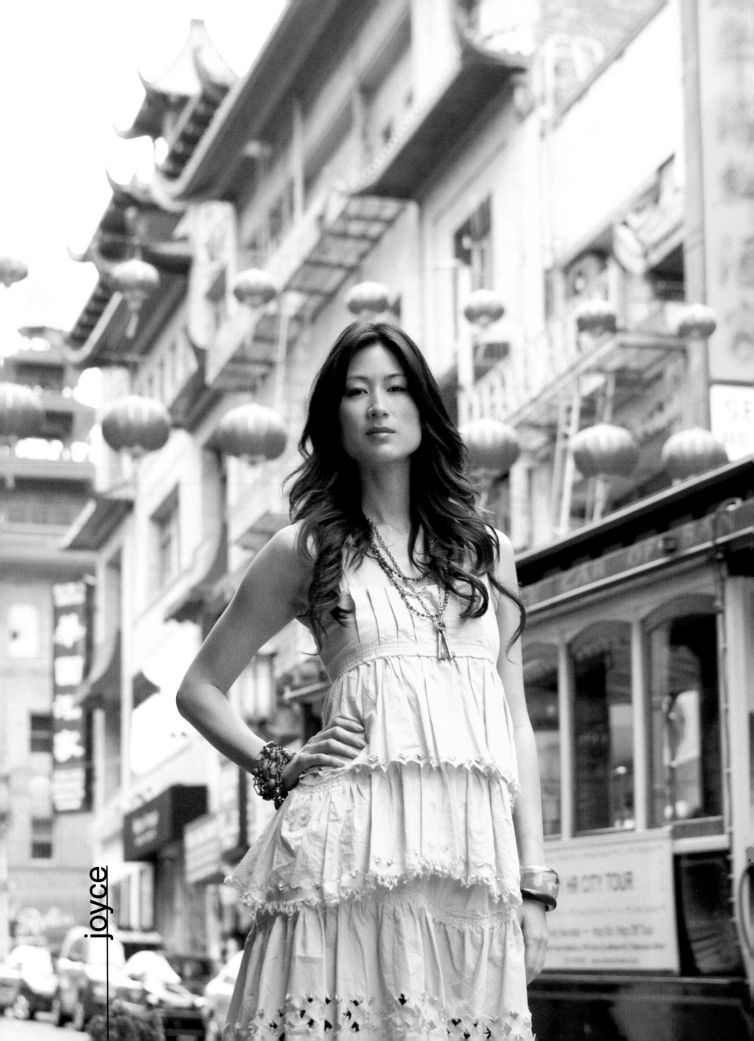

joyce

# san francisco

*The day we arrived in San Francisco it was raining and we were told it had been raining for months straight, but even through the veil of water the city was very fashionable. I call the San Francisco style bohemian chic, and it really stands out from other cities. Blame it on San Francisco being the center of the hippie culture in the 1960s; I believe the style still resonates there. Makeup here is secondary to great hair and clothes so keep it fresh and simple. Look for gold and bronze tones with creamy sheer lip colors like brick or pink.*

1  Apply a highlight stick foundation to the center of the face.
2  Blend in a contour foundation a shade darker to the outside of the face.
3  Apply under-eye concealer where necessary.
4  Apply dark brown brow pencil to brows.
5  Use a cream gold eye shadow at base.
6  Apply dark brown pencil eyeliner.
7  Apply black mascara.
8  Apply three-quarter lashes.
9  Apply bronze cream blush to apples of cheeks to temples.
10  Apply warm brown lip liner.
11  Apply sheer cool brick lipstick.

## focal points

Use a **dark brown brow pencil** at ends of brows to create definition. Apply a **gold cream highlighter** to base of lid. Apply **dark brown liner** on top and bottom lash line from the center of the pupil to the end corners of the eyes. Curl upper lashes and apply **black mascara** to the top and bottom lashes. Apply **three-quarter strip lashes** from the ends first and as close to the lash line as possible. Concentrating on the end corners of the eyes gives the illusion of wider eyes creating more symmetry to her face.

Use a **warm brown lip liner** to define the natural lip line. Apply a **sheer cool brick lip color**.

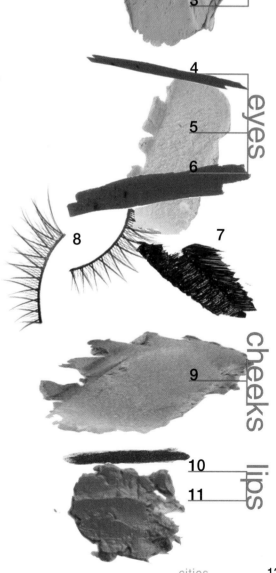

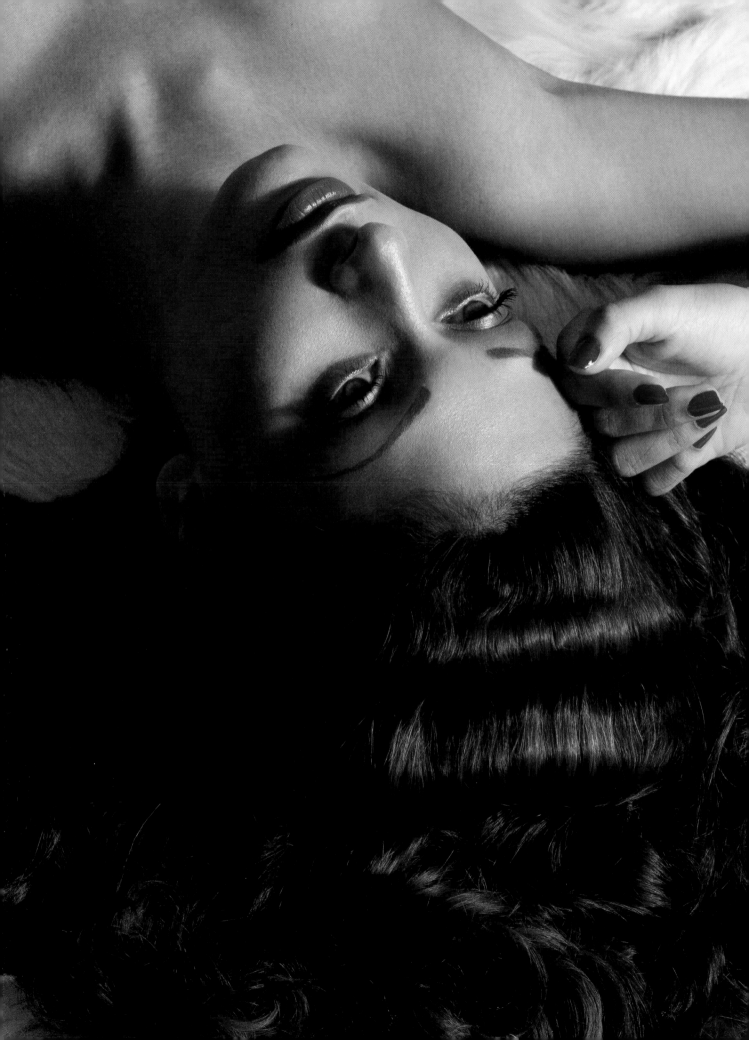

I LOVE THE '60s and '70s. Even as a little girl watching movies like *Grease* and *Saturday Night Fever*, I was obsessed with Sandy's makeover and still remember it so vividly to this day. What happened to old Hollywood glamour queens like Marlena Dietrich, Joan Crawford, and Sophia Loren? Why have I never seen these fantastic decade looks on Asian women with the exception of Suzi Wong? These were questions that I had for years. I was ecstatic to finally do Asian versions of the period looks I so admired but had never seen. This is what this chapter is all about.

Fashion continuously borrows from these decades every season, so whether you dress in period looks on a daily basis (cheers to you!) or just want to try it for fun, learn to take bits and pieces of these highly stylized looks to get your own decades-inspired look.

# decades

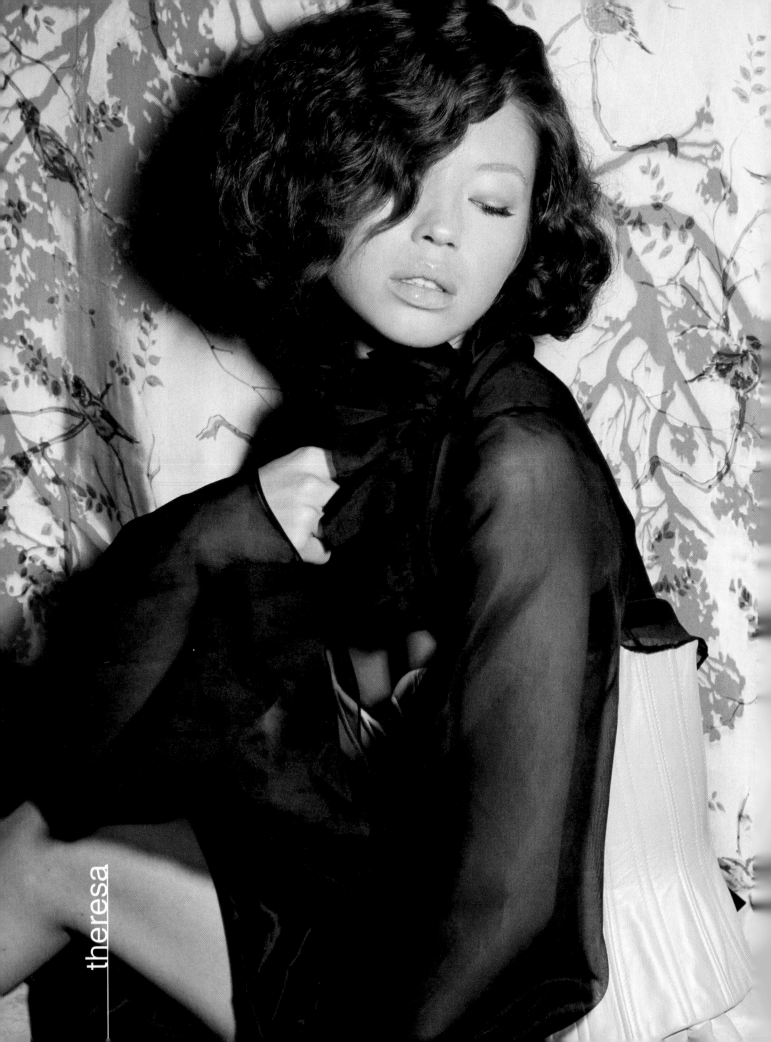

theresa

1. Apply a highlight foundation to the center of the face.
2. Blend in a contour foundation to the outside of the face.
3. Apply under-eye concealer where necessary.
4. Use a darker concealer for the skin.
5. Set with translucent powder.
6. Apply ash brown brow cream to brows.
7. Apply darker concealer on lids.
8. Apply eye gloss.
9. Apply black mascara.
10. Apply individual black lashes.
11. Apply pale warm pink blush to apples of cheeks.
12. Apply concealer.
13. Apply clear lip gloss.

## focal points

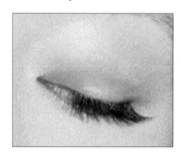

Use contour **foundation** or concealer to create natural-looking depth on the eyelid. Curl lashes, apply **black mascara**, and add **short black individual lashes** on the outer corners. Using a **large lip or concealer brush** carefully apply eye gloss. Be careful not to apply too close to the lash line.

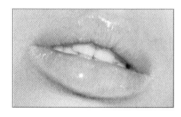

Apply **concealer** on the entire mouth, blending well into the mouth area. (You can also use **nude lip gloss**, similar to your skin tone.) Apply **clear lip gloss**.

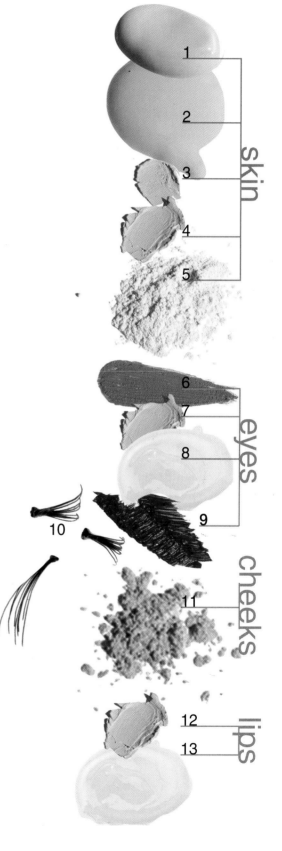

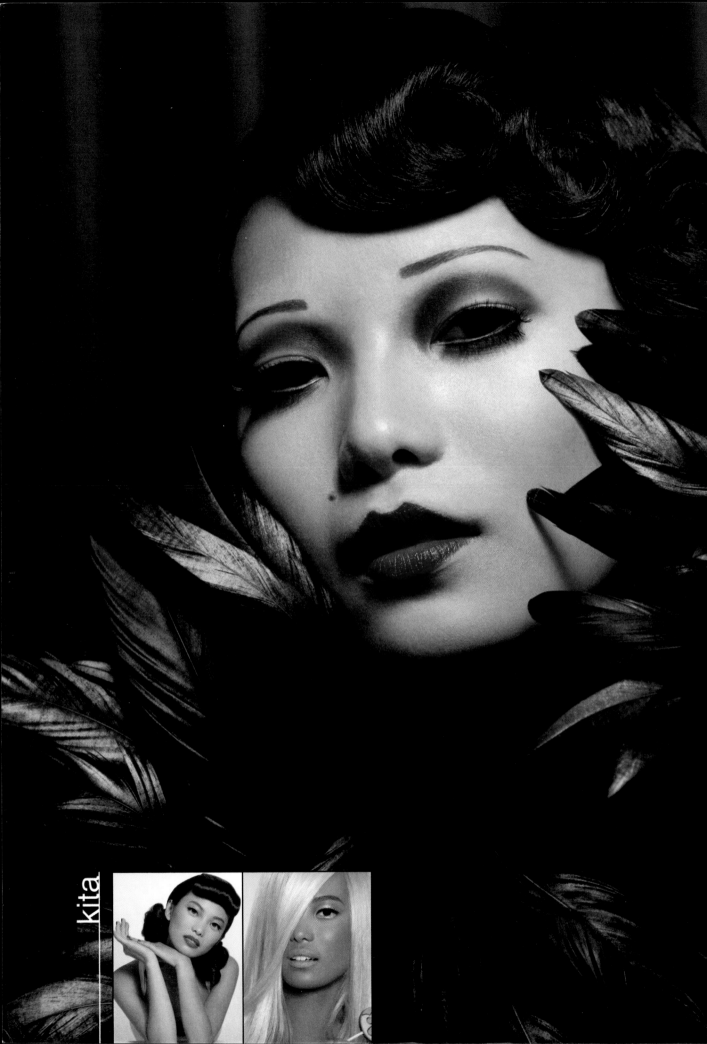

kita

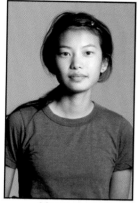

**kita before**

1. Apply sealer wax to brows.
2. Set with brow wax sealer.
3. Apply a highlight foundation to the center of the face.
4. Blend in a contour foundation to the outside of the face and contour nose.
5. Apply concealer where necessary and use to cover natural lip line.
6. Use a darker concealer for the skin.
7. Set with translucent powder.
8. Apply dark ash brown brow cream to brows.
9. Use dark brown shadow.
10. Apply black eye shadow.
11. Apply black eyeliner.
12. Apply white eyeliner.
13. Apply black mascara.
14. Apply full strip eyelashes.
15. Apply bottom strip eyelashes.
16. Apply black liquid eyeliner.
17. Apply blush to apples of cheeks.
18. Apply lip balm.
19. Apply dark fig lip liner.

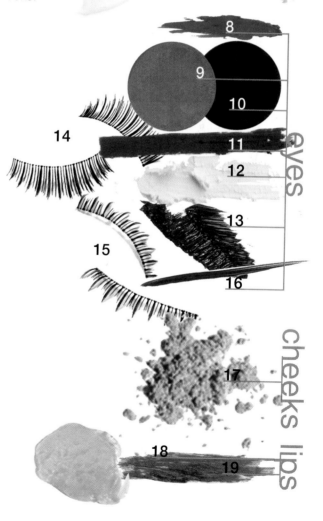

## focal points

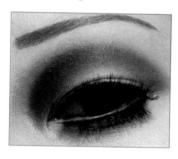

Apply **sealer wax** to eyebrows. Set wax using **brow wax sealer**. Allow to dry for a couple minutes. Apply **concealer** over waxed area. Use a **dark brown shadow** to contour the eyelid (the top rim of layer 2). I created an even more intense depth using a touch of **black shadow** on the inner corners. Apply a thin line of **black eyeliner** along the top and bottom lash line. Apply **white eyeliner** inside the lower rim. Curl lashes and apply **black mascara** to the top and bottom lashes. Apply **full strip eyelashes** to the top lashes and then apply the **bottom strip eyelashes**. Cover any remaining glue with **black liquid eyeliner**. Add more mascara if necessary.

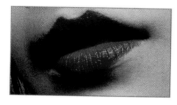

Make sure lips are hydrated using **lip balm**. Remove any excess with tissue. Use **concealer** to erase natural lip line. Use **dark fig lip liner** to create a new small bow-like shape and fill in to create a dark matte lip.

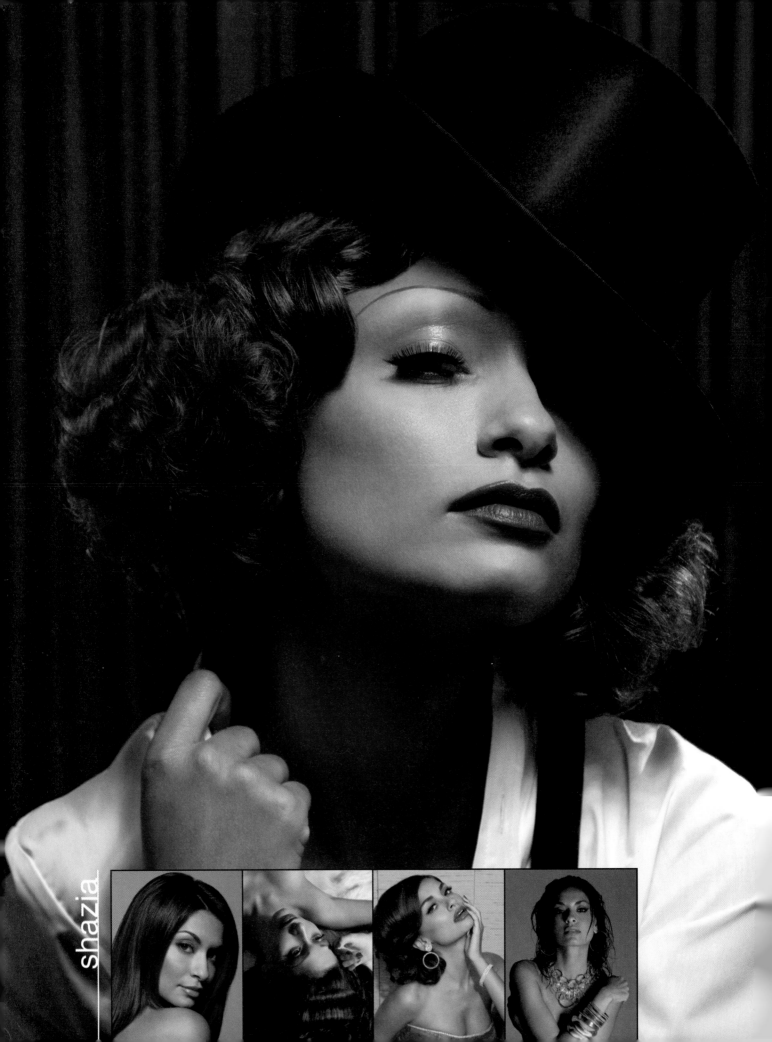

shazia

1 Apply sealer wax to brows.
2 Set with brow wax sealer.
3 Apply a highlight foundation to the center of the face.
4 Blend in a contour foundation to the outside of the face and lids.
5 Apply concealer under eyes and on waxed brows.
6 Set with translucent yellow-based loose powder.
7 Apply brown eyebrow pencil to brows.
8 Apply clear gloss at base.
9 Apply black mascara.
10 Apply full strip eyelashes.
11 Apply black liquid eyeliner.
12 Apply bronzer along cheekbones.
13 Apply warm brick lip pencil.
14 Apply brick matte lipstick.

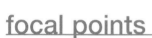

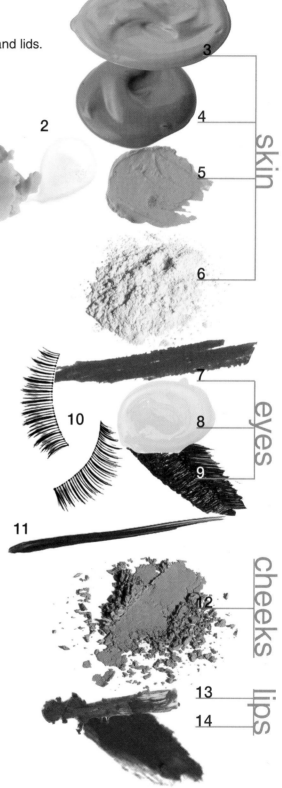

**skin**

**eyes**

**cheeks**

**lips**

## focal points

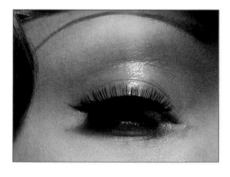

Apply **sealer wax** to eyebrows. Set wax using **brow wax sealer**. Allow to dry for a couple minutes. Apply **concealer** over waxed area. Use **contour foundation** on base of lid to add depth naturally (layer 2), then apply **clear gloss** over the contoured area (layer 2). Draw in a thin rounded eyebrow using a **dark brown eyebrow pencil**. Apply **full strip of eyelashes**. Apply **black liquid eyeliner** along the lash line and create a thin wing at outer corners.

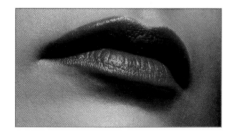

Overdraw the top lip using a **warm brick lip pencil**, creating wide peaks. Line entire mouth. Blend over liner a **creamy brick-colored lipstick**.

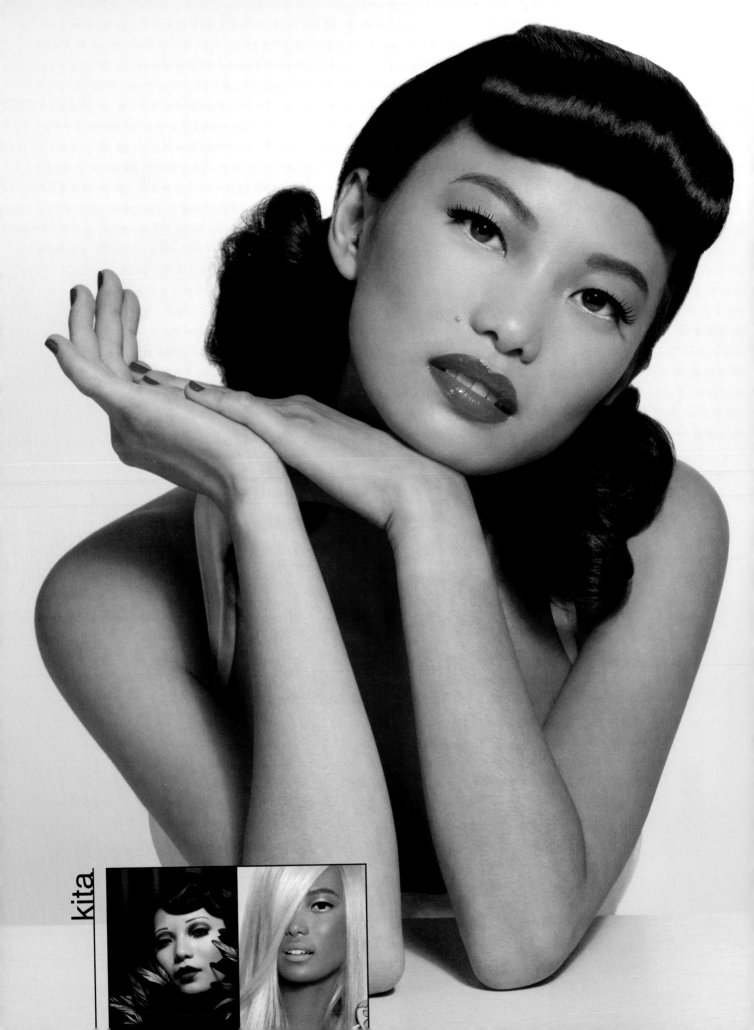

kita.

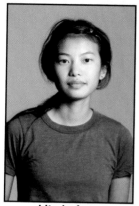

**kita before**

1 Apply cream foundation all over face.
2 Blend in a contour foundation under cheekbones and on eyelids.
3 Apply a cake eye concealer under eyes.
4 Set with shimmery powder.
5 Apply ash brown brow cream to brows.
6 Curl lashes and apply mascara to top lashes only.
7 Apply full set of eyelashes.
8 Use a black liquid eyeliner along the lash line.
9 Apply mascara again onto false lashes.
10 Apply white liner along the inside rim.
11 Apply pale pink blush to apples of cheeks.
12 Apply cream highlighter above apples and at temples.
13 Apply a bright pink lipstick.
14 Finish the look with a clear lip gloss.

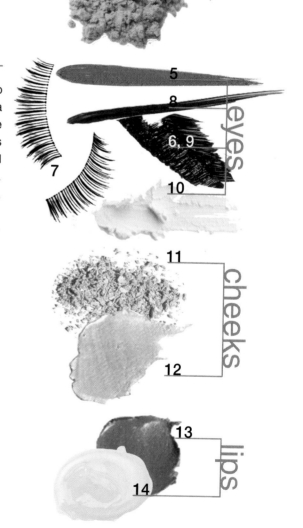

skin

## focal points

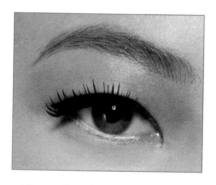

**white eyeliner** inside the lower rim.

Use a **warm cream brown liner** to create a full angled brow. Apply a **contouring foundation** over entire lid. This adds depth to the eyes without adding color. Curl natural lashes and apply **black mascara**. Apply **full strip false eyelashes**, adding more mascara if necessary. Apply **black liquid eyeliner** along the lash line. Finish the look with

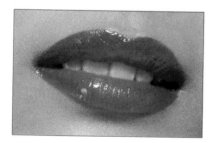

Apply a **bright pink cream lipstick** using a **lip brush** to create a full mouth. Apply a **clear lip gloss to the center of the mouth** to create a sexy pout.

eyes

cheeks

lips

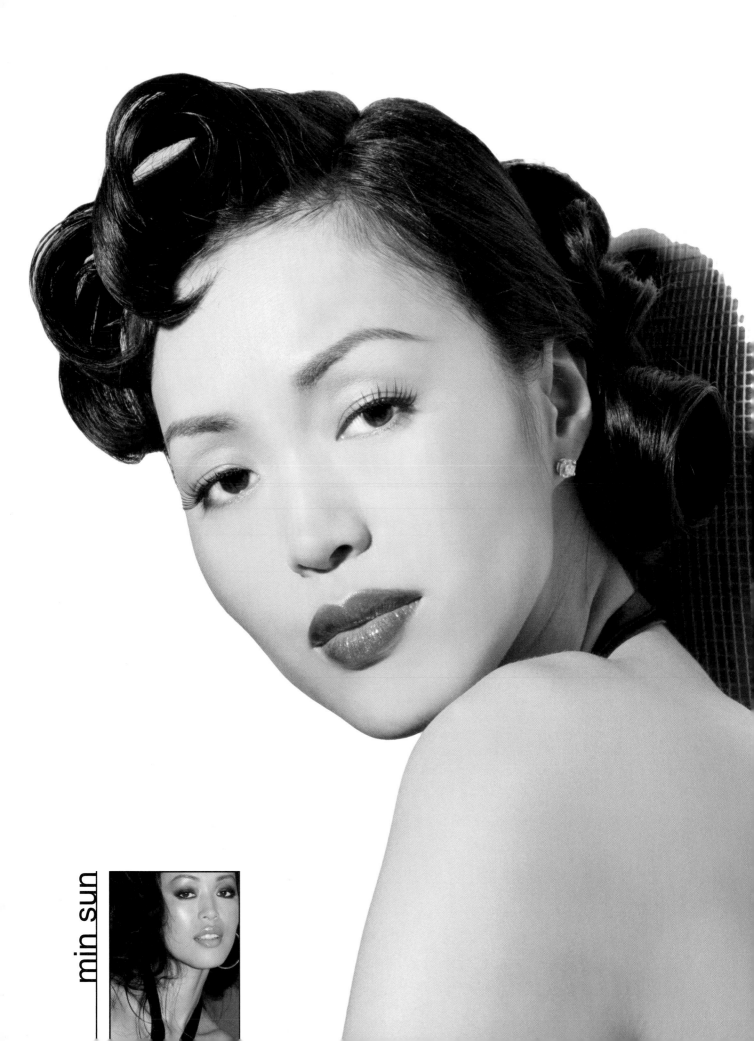

min sun

# 1940s sophisticate

1. Apply liquid foundation all over the face.
2. Apply under-eye concealer.
3. Set with sheer loose powder.
4. Apply ash brown brow cream.
5. Apply warm pink eye shadow at base.
6. Apply black liquid eyeliner.
7. Curl lashes, then apply black mascara to top and bottom lashes.
8. Apply full set of false eyelashes.
9. Apply soft pink blush to apples of cheeks and temples.
10. Apply cream highlighter above apples and temples.
11. Apply lip balm.
12. Apply warm brown lip liner.
13. Apply deep berry lip gloss.

## focal points

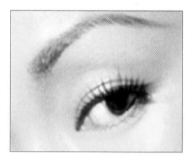

Create a perfectly angled brow using an **angle brow brush** and an **ash brown brow pomade**. Concentrate more color at the end of brows. Apply a **warm pink shadow** to base of lid (layer 2). Apply a thin line of **black liquid eyeliner** along the lash line finishing it with a 45- degree angle at the end of the eye. Curl lashes and apply **black mascara** to top and bottom lashes. Apply a **full set of false eyelashes**.

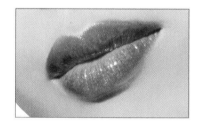

Apply **lip balm**. Line lips gently using **warm brown lip liner** adding a few strokes to the center of the lower lips. Gently rub together and fill in with a **deep berry lip gloss** or lip color.

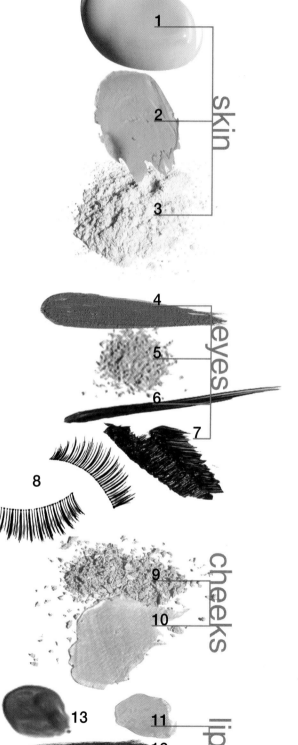

skin
1
2
3

eyes
4
5
6
7
8

cheeks
9
10

lips
13
11
12

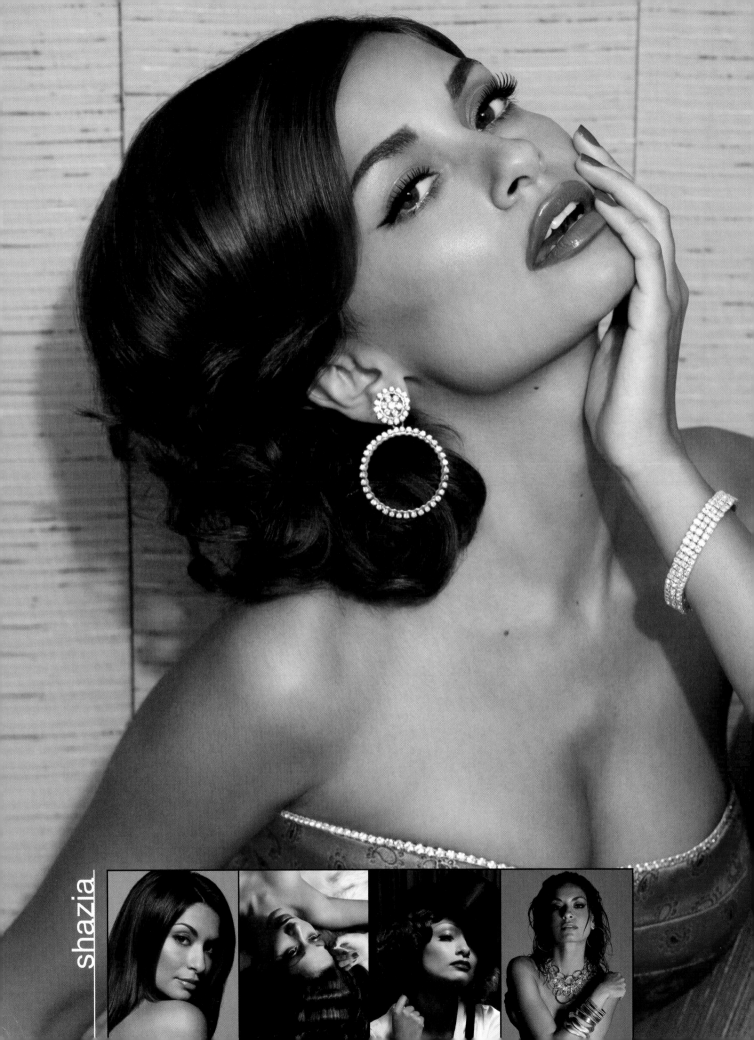

shazia

1 Apply a highlight foundation to the center of the face.
2 Blend in a contour foundation to the outside of the face.
3 Apply under-eye concealer where necessary.
4 Set with shimmery sheer golden brown loose powder.
5 Apply brown brow cream to brows.
6 Apply chestnut brown eye shadow.
7 Apply black eyeliner.
8 Apply white eyeliner.
9 Apply black mascara.
10 Apply full strip false lashes.
11 Apply black liquid eyeliner.
12 Apply bronzer along cheekbones.
13 Apply shimmery sheer golden brown loose powder above apples and at temples.
14 Apply neutral lip liner.
15 Apply warm pink lip gloss.

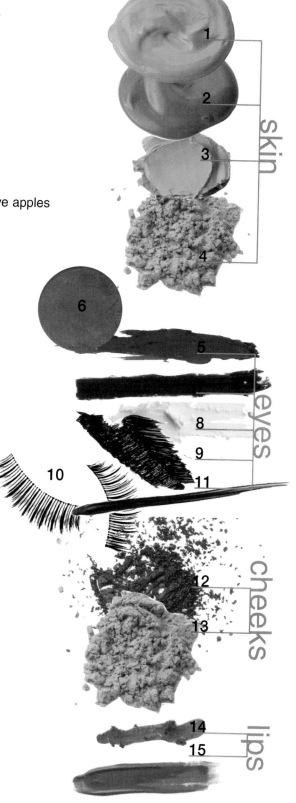

skin

eyes

cheeks

lips

## focal points

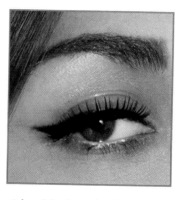

Apply **brown brow cream** to brows creating a full squared brow. Apply **chestnut brown shadow** along the base of the lid and the lower lash line. Create a winged eye using a thick line of **black eyeliner**. Apply **white pencil eyeliner** inside lower rims. Curl lashes, apply **black mascara** to top and bottom lashes. Apply **full strip of lashes**. Apply **black liquid liner** to the top lash line and over black pencil line to create a sharper edge.

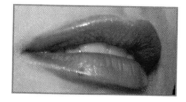

Create a fuller mouth using **neutral lip liner** around the natural lip line. Apply a **warm rose-colored creamy lipstick** over entire mouth.

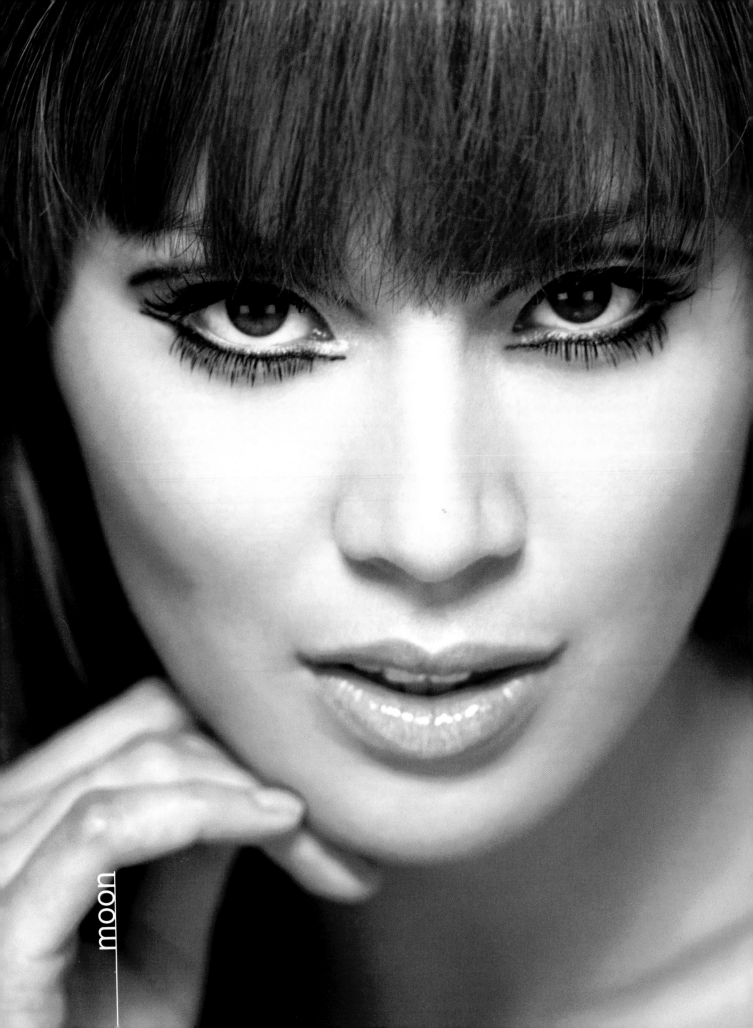

moon

*Moon is one of the big inspirations behind this book. I met her on a photo shoot and she has been incredibly supportive ever since. She is such an amazing talent and I am blessed to have her in my life. Moon took Hollywood by storm and shares the spotlight on the small and big screens with some of Hollywood's finest actors and is also an amazing singer and songwriter.*

1  Apply illuminating lotion.
2  Apply a highlight foundation to the center of the face.
3  Blend in a contour foundation to the outside of the face.
4  Apply under-eye concealer where necessary.
5  Set with translucent yellow-based powder.
6  Apply neutral brown brow cream to brows.
7  Use a white shimmery eye shadow.
8  Apply black eyeliner.
9  Apply black mascara.
10  Apply full strip eyelashes.
11  Apply full lower lash strip.
12  Apply black liquid eyeliner.
13  Apply pale pink blush to apples of cheeks.
14  Apply cream highlighter above apples and at temples.
15  Apply concealer.
16  Apply clear lip gloss.

## focal points

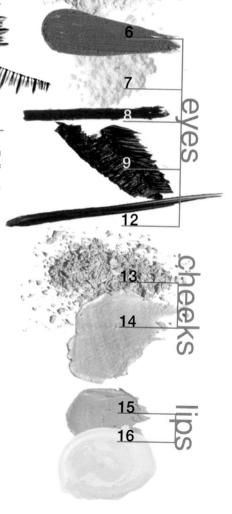

skin

eyes

cheeks

lips

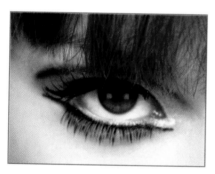

Apply **white shimmery eye shadow** on the base of lids and along inner corners of the eye. Use a **black eyeliner pencil** to draw a curved line above the entire eye. (Make sure it's high enough that when you open your eyes you still see a lot of white lid space.) Apply a thick line of **black eyeliner** along the top and bottom lash line, extending out the ends (but not connecting). Curl lashes and apply **black mascara**. Apply **full set of eyelashes** to the top lid and full lower lash strip to the bottom lash line. Apply **black liquid liner** to create any sharp lines (lower lash line) and extended ends. Apply **white eyeliner** inside lower rims.

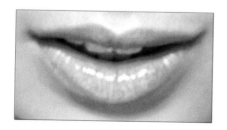

Apply **concealer** over entire mouth, blending well into the surrounding skin. (Some concealers can be too drying, You can substitute concealer for **nude lip gloss**.) Apply **clear lip gloss** to complete the look.

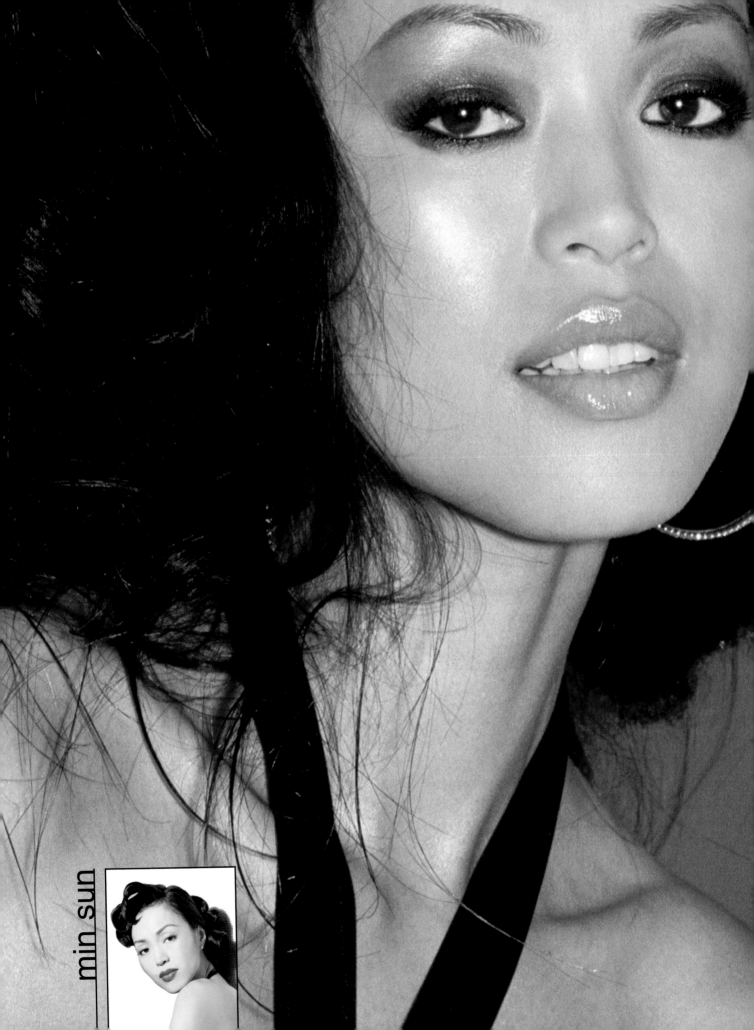

min sun

1  Apply a highlight foundation to the center of the face.
2  Blend in a contour foundation to the outside of the face.
3  Apply under-eye concealer where necessary.
4  Set with sheer yellow-based powder powder.
5  Apply ash brown brow cream to brows.
6  Use a plum-colored eye shadow at base.
7  Apply light copper shadow at brow bone.
8  Apply black eye shadow.
9  Apply black eyeliner.
10  Apply black mascara.
11  Apply full set black lashes.
12  Apply black liquid eyeliner.
13  Apply pale pink blush to apples of cheeks.
14  Apply cream highlighter above apples and at temples.
15  Apply neutral lip liner.
16  Apply pink shimmery lip gloss.

## focal points

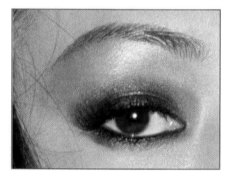

Use an **ash brown brow cream** using an angled brow brush and concentrating on the end of the brows. Use a **dark plum eye shadow** at the base of the lid (layer 2). Apply a light **copper shadow** under brow bone (layer 1). Apply **black eye shadow** around entire eye (layer 3). Apply **black eyeliner** around entire eye. Apply **black eyeliner** inside lower rim. Curl lashes and apply **black mascara** to the top and bottom lashes. Apply **full strip of black false eyelashes**.

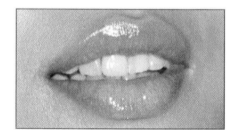

Use a **neutral-colored lip liner** to create a perfectly symmetrical lip and also to accentuate the outline. Apply a few strokes in the center to create a blend. Use a **shimmery pink lip gloss** to blend together.

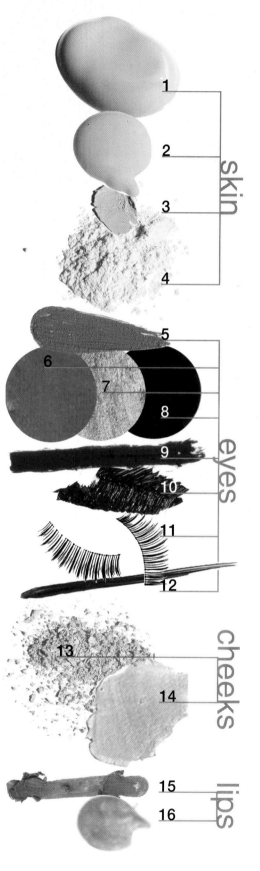

skin

eyes

cheeks

lips

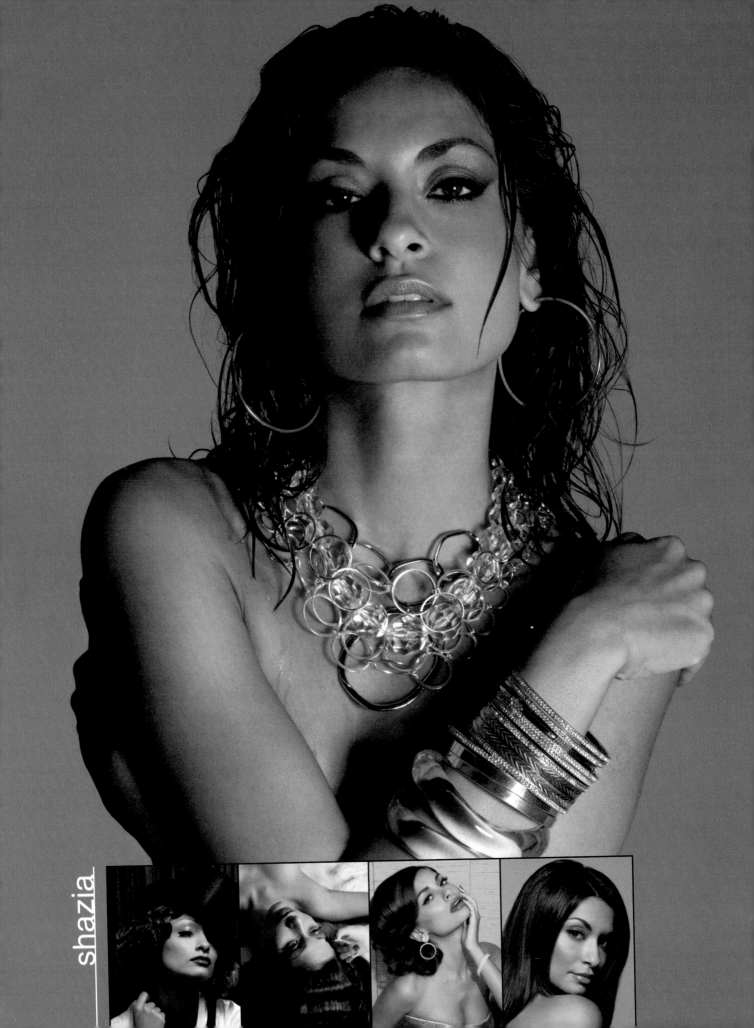

shazia.

1. Apply a highlight foundation to the center of the face.
2. Blend in a contour foundation to the outside of the face.
3. Apply under-eye concealer where necessary.
4. Set with translucent yellow-based powder.
5. Apply ash brown brow cream to brows.
6. Use a pink cream eye shadow.
7. Use lavender cream eye shadow.
8. Apply black eyeliner.
9. Apply black mascara.
10. Apply short individual lashes.
11. Apply pink blush along the cheekbones.
12. Apply lip balm.
13. Apply pale purple lipstick.

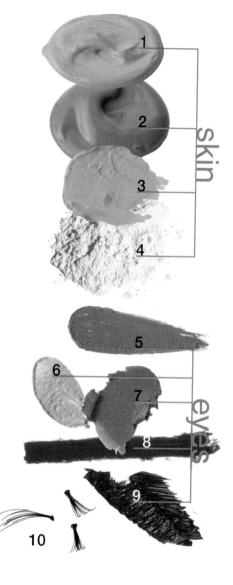

skin

eyes

cheeks

lips

## focal points

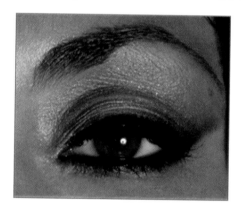

Apply **ashy brown brow cream** to ends of brows. Apply **pink cream eye shadow** to brow bone and layer 3. Apply **lavender cream shadow** to layer 2 (in crease only) and along bottom lash line. Apply **black eyeliner** around entire eye, winging out the outer corners. Apply **black eyeliner** inside the lower lash line. Curl lashes and apply **black mascara** to both top and bottom lashes. Apply a few **individual lashes** to the outer corners.

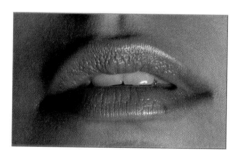

Apply **lip balm** to lips. Apply **creamy shimmery pale purple** lipstick over entire mouth.

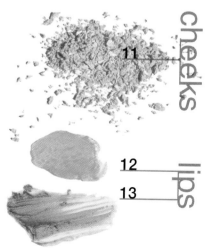

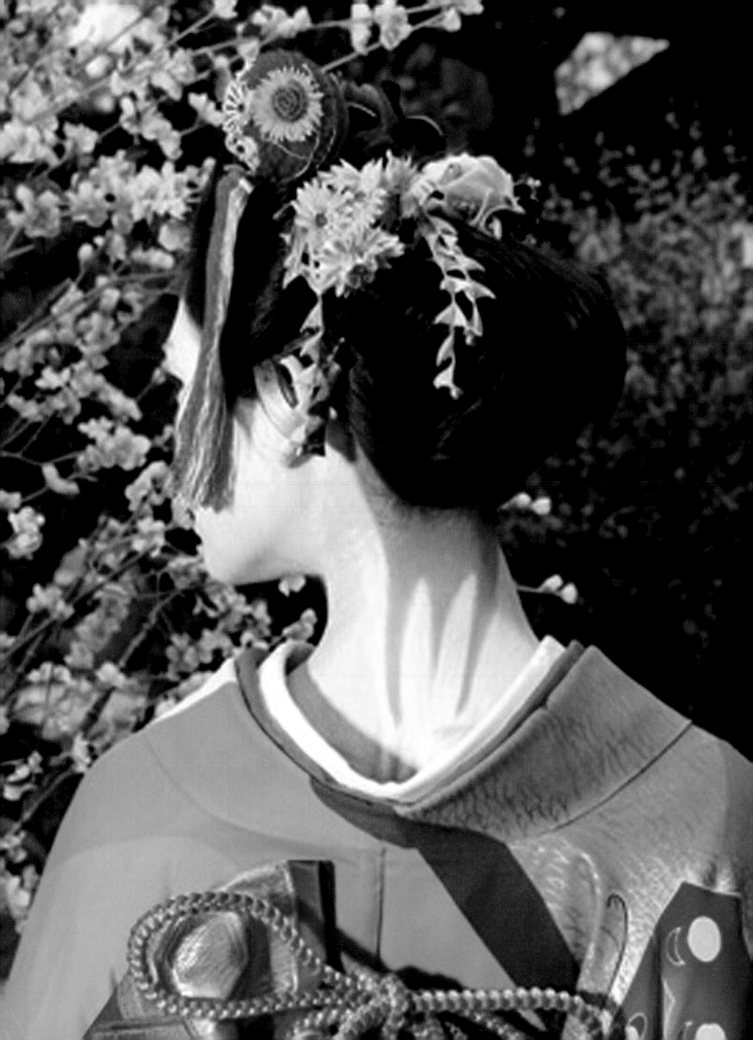

ALMOST EVERY YEAR I go to a costume party. I always look forward to dressing up and enjoy the chance to become someone else for a night. I plan my often outrageous outfit weeks in advance. It's fun and exciting to play a new role and makeup completes the transformation. It continues to amaze me how with just the flick of a brush, you can go back in time and experience what it feels like to be a geisha with a painted face, or bring back a classic style movement like the Goth trend. And when you nail the look, the right attitude always follows! With these more complex makeup applications, practice makes perfect, so as always, don't be discouraged if it takes a couple of tries before you achieve the look you want.

# costume

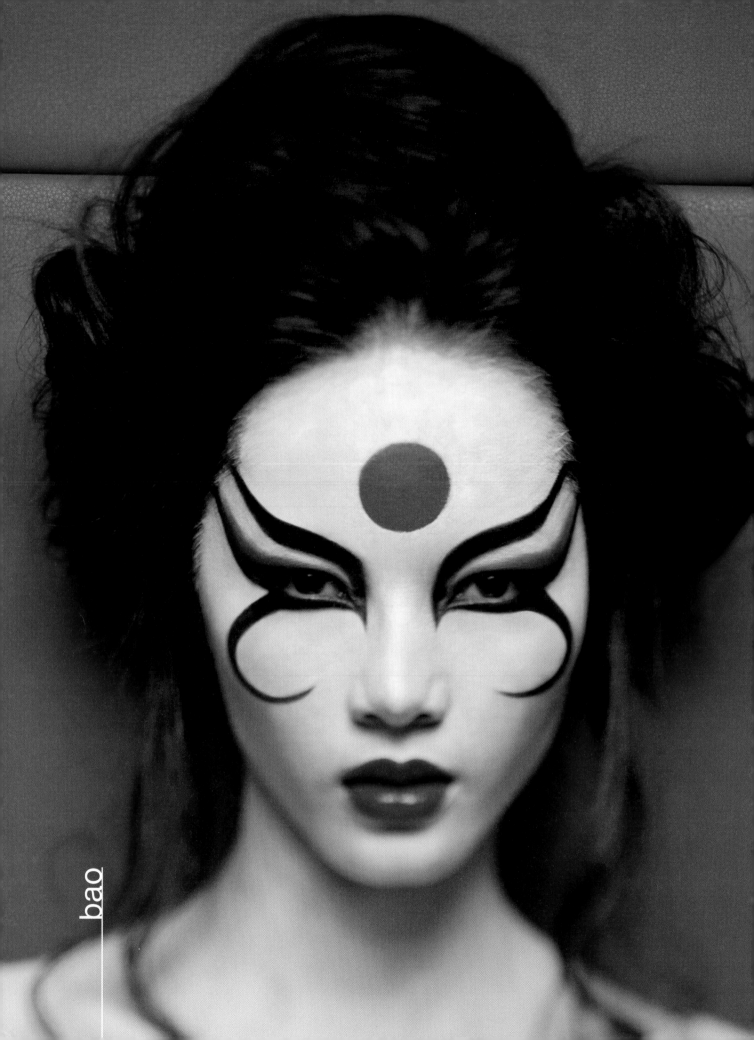

bao

# modern kabuki

*Kabuki means "song, dance, and skill." This very stylized theatrical performance was started by a woman, but is now actually performed only by men. They even play the female parts. The marks and colors on the faces describe the character, whether they're heroes or villains. I love the intensity and beauty it creates.*

1 Apply sealer wax to brows.
2 Set with brow wax sealer.
3 Apply black eyeliner.
4 Apply black cream shadow or paint.
5 Apply white face base.
6 Apply purple eye shadow.
7 Apply white eyeliner.
8 Apply black mascara.
9 Mix white face paint with moisturizer.
10 Set with white powder.
11 Apply red face paint.
12 Apply red lipstick.

**Cool Tip**
Use white cream foundation with a concealer brush as an eraser to fix any mistakes. Make sure to clean excess off the brush.

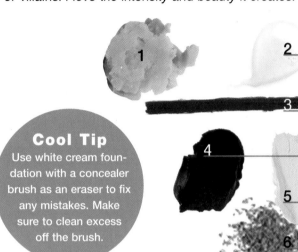

## focal points

Start by using **black liner** to draw out the shape of the eye, then fill in with **black cream eye shadow or paint**. I did this freehand but you can also use **stencils**, then use the **white foundation** and a **concealer brush** to clean up any mistakes and fill in blank areas on lids and temples. Follow with some **purple shadow** to add color following the top of the black line on the eyelid. Use **white liner** on the inside lower lids and apply **black mascara** to finish the look.

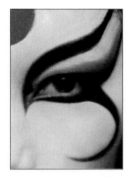

Mix **white cream foundation** with **moisturizer** and apply to all exposed skin and mouth using a **foundation brush**. Use **concealer brush** for the hard-to-reach areas and to clean up mistakes. Set with white powder using a **small powder brush**.

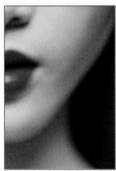

Make sure there is no white on lips and fill in with **cherry red lipstick**. Use a brush for better precision.

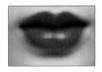

Create an empty circle by cleaning off white base on forehead using a **cotton swab** and **makeup remover**. Fill in with **red face paint**.

**Bao in Kabuki makeup, inspired by the book *Kabuki* by David Mack.**

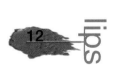

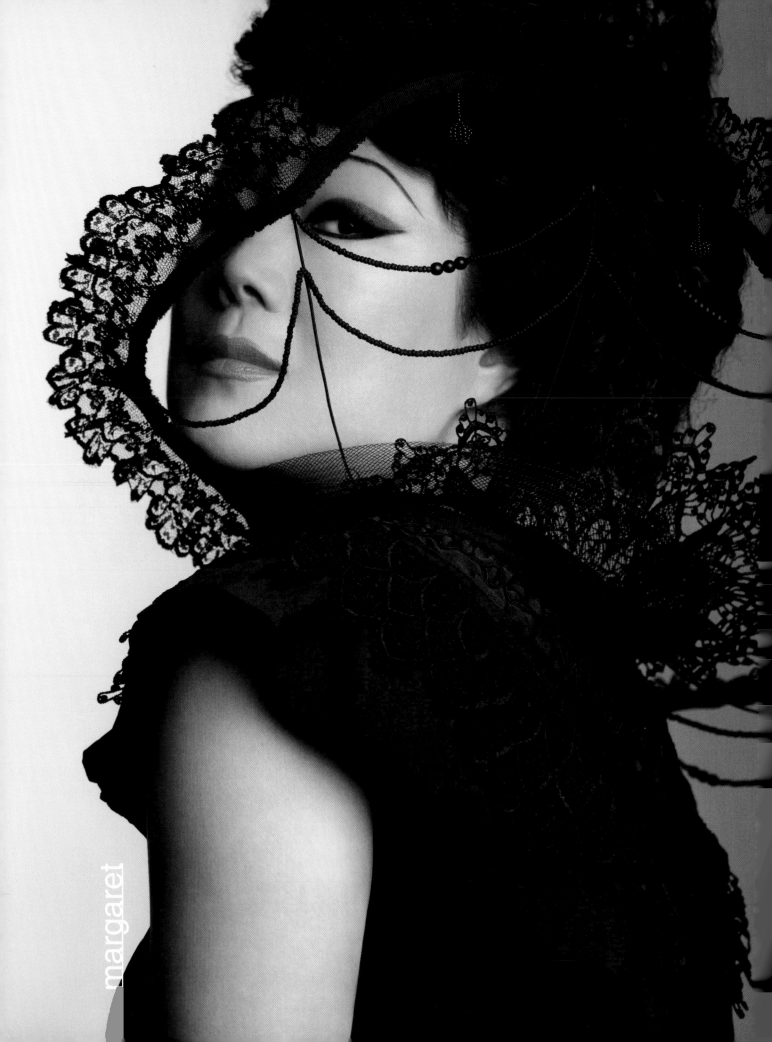

margaret

# dark victorian

*This look is a slight twist on the goth subculture that is prevalent in so many countries. I clearly remember this "dark" look during the '80s in many bands. The goth look is usually associated with black clothes and makeup. Victorian clothes began to be used as the clothing styles of goth, but you can still find different versions of the goth look almost everywhere.*

1. Apply sealer wax to brows.
2. Set with brow wax sealer.
3. Mix foundation with some white makeup base to make the skin a couple shades lighter.
4. Apply concealer where necessary, especially brows.
5. Set with translucent powder.
6. Apply black eye brow pencil.
7. Apply black eyeliner.
8. Apply dark brown cream eye shadow.
9. Apply black mascara.
10. Apply full strip false eyelashes.
11. Apply black liquid eyeliner.
12. Apply beige pink blush at apples.
13. Apply neutral lip liner.
14. Apply bright true orange cream lipstick.

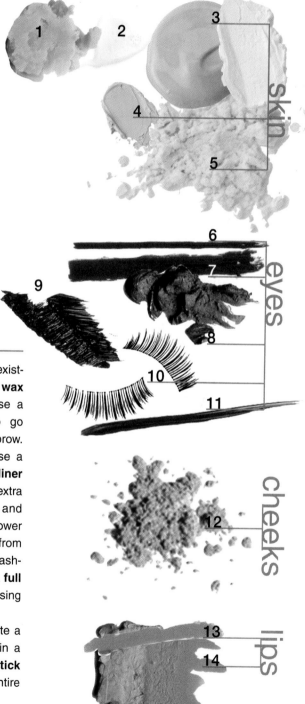

## focal points

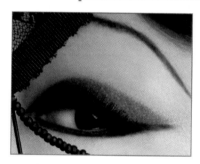

Apply **brow wax** to conceal existing eyebrows. Set with **brow wax sealer** and allow to dry. Use a **black eyebrow pencil** to go along the topline of the eyebrow. Leave the brows natural. Use a thick line of **black pencil eyeliner** to wing out the eyes. Apply extra along the top lash line and smudge up to create a thick line. Apply **black eyeliner** inside the lower rim. Apply **dark brown cream shadow** above the black line starting from the middle of the eye and following through to the winged tip. Curl lashes and apply **black mascara** on the top and bottom lashes. Apply a **full strip of false lashes** on the top lashes. Cover up any glue lines using **black liquid eyeliner**.

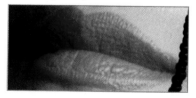

Use **neutral lip liner** to create a slightly larger mouth. Blend in a **bright orange cream lipstick** over the liner and fill in the entire mouth.

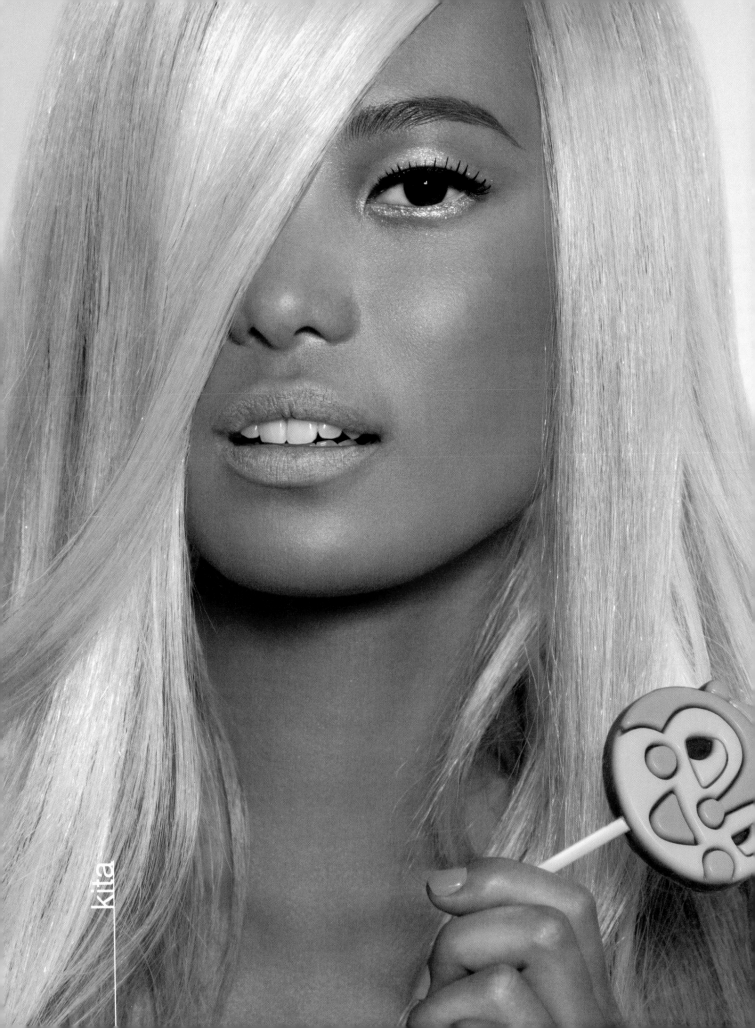

kita

# ganguro

This is a toned-down version of the over-the-top Ganguro fashion trend that began in Tokyo. The style consists of contrasts and colors—bleached hair, dark skin, pale lips, white and black liner, shimmery shadows, and colorful clothes. I love the Ganguro girls' boldness, and it's evident that they really have fun with their look.

1 Apply a highlight foundation to the center of the face several shades darker than your natural skin tone but lighter than contouring color. (Self tanner is also widely used.)
2 Blend in a contour bronzing foundation to the outside of the face, eyelids, neck, and chest.
3 Apply under-eye concealer.
4 Set with golden shimmery loose powder.
5 Apply ash brown brow cream to brows.
6 Use a creamy champagne liner on base of eyelid.
7 Use white eyeliner inside lower rim of eye.
8 Apply white metallic shadow under eyes along lash line and inner corners.
9 Apply black mascara.
10 Apply full strip false eyelashes.
11 Apply black eyeliner.
12 Apply bronzer along the cheekbone.
13 Apply concealer on lips.
14 Apply pale pink lipstick.

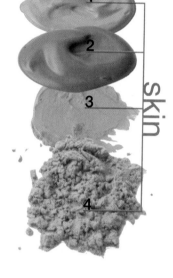

## focal points

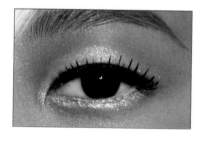

Apply a **champagne cream eyeliner** on base of lid. Apply **white eyeliner** inside the lower rim and apply **white metallic eye shadow** along the lower lash line and inner corners of the eyes. Apply **extra white metallic shadow** along the base of the top lid to add more shimmer. Apply **black mascara** on top lashes only. Apply a **full strip of eyelashes**. Finish off with **black liquid eyeliner** along the top lash line.

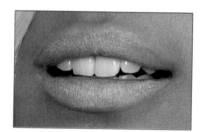

Use **concealer** to neutralize natural lip color. Apply **pale pink lipstick** over entire mouth.

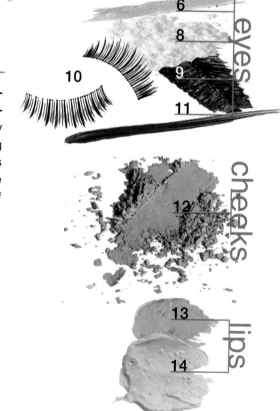

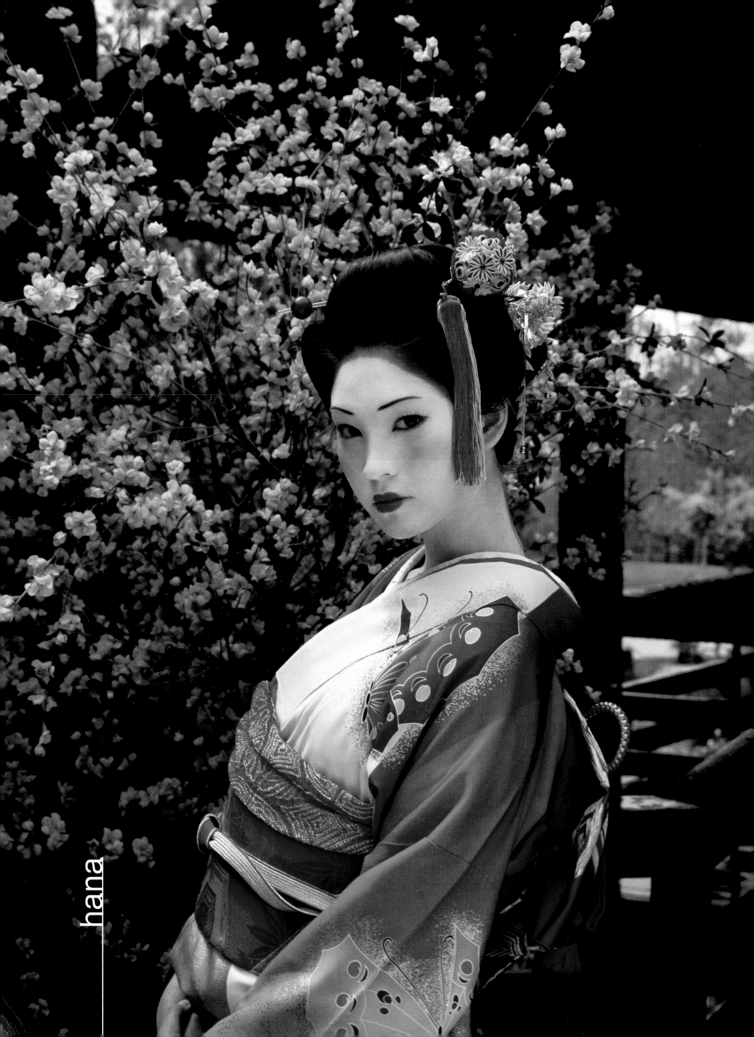

hana

# geisha

*Geisha means "art person." Geishas study many forms of performance art, including several dances, singing, and instruments, as well as the art of conversation and serving. Girls train to be Maiko (apprentice geisha) from a very young age and after up to six years they have the chance to become Geiko (full-fledged geisha). You can tell the difference between maiko and geisha mostly by their clothing and hair ornaments. The maiko wear brightly colored kimonos as well as hair ornaments. The geisha have more subdued kimonos and usually only wear a simple comb in their hair.*
*Both are incredibly beautiful.*

1 Apply sealer wax to brows.
2 Set with brow wax sealer.
3+4 Mix moisturizer with white foundation base.
5 Set with white loose powder.
6 Apply black pencil for brows.
7 Apply pink eyeliner pencil.
8 Apply black liquid eyeliner.
9 Apply black mascara.
10 Apply blush to apples of cheeks beginning under the pupil.
11 Apply cherry red cream lipstick.

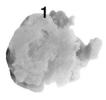

### Cool Tip
Use white cream foundation with a concealer brush as an eraser to fix any mistakes. Make sure to clean excess off the brush.

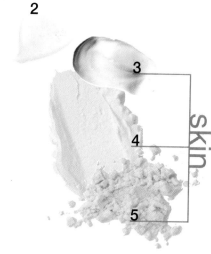

skin

## focal points

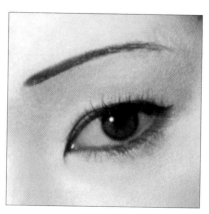

Apply **brow wax** to conceal existing eyebrows. Set with **brow wax sealer** and allow to dry. Mix **white foundation base mixed with moisturizer** and apply all over face, including eyelids and mouth, up to but not into the hairline. Set with **white loose powder**. Draw a thin flat brow above natural brows using a **black eyeliner pencil**. Apply **pink eyeliner pencil** along top lid and lower bottom corner. Apply a thin line of **black liquid eyeliner** along the top lash line. Curl lashes and apply **black mascara** to top and bottom lashes

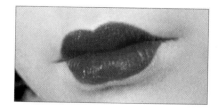

Conceal the natural lip line using a **white base**. Apply a **creamy cherry red lipstick** to create a rounded pouty mouth.

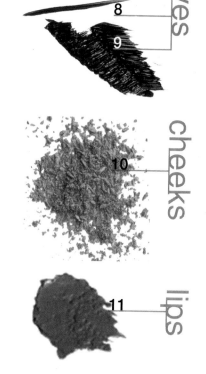

eyes

cheeks

lips

# acknowledgments

First and foremost I want to thank God for all of his blessings. I am amazed every day how much I've grown, and I am grateful for the past, good and bad, which has made me who I am today.

Words cannot express how honored and grateful I am to Yoko Ono. Thank you for your kind words and support. I continue to be amazed by your generosity and kindness.

All my love and thanks to the best literary agent ever, Melissa Flashman at Trident Media Group, who believed in this book from day one and took it from an idea to reality. You held my hand throughout the whole thing. I will be forever grateful for your support and belief in me.

To everyone at Perigee: Jeanette Shaw, thank you for your tireless efforts and patience and for taking on this project and being truly encouraging and supportive. Tiffany Estreicher, thank you for your patience, kindness, and all that you taught me through this process. Thanks to my publisher, John Duff. Kellie Schirmer, Pauline Neuwirth, and Charles Bjorklund, thank you for your work on this book that is so near and dear to my heart. Thank you for being a part of a dream come true.

To Christel Winkler, thank you for believing in this book and truly getting it. Your positive energy and excitement really helped push me through.

To everyone at the Cloutier Agency: Chantal Cloutier, thank you for the honor of being a part of such an amazing team. Madeline Leonard, who I respect incredibly and put on the highest pedestal. We started with scraps and drawings and here we are. Cheers to you for your relentless support. To Charnelle Smith, thank you for giving me my staff. Jill Shillaw, thank you for always being on it and continuing to make me soar. Brooke Bryant, thank you for pushing me and rooting for me. To Adrienne, Toni, Corey, Suzi, Heather, and Jessica, thank you for your support system, for your smiles and constant help with everything. To Kim Goodwin, Gwen Kellet, Heather Currie, Natasha Stanford Lerch, and everyone at Cloutier past and present. All of you took me in with nothing and believed in me. Thank you for pushing me and building me on a daily basis. I would not be here today without all of you.

Undying gratitude to everyone who believed in this book and went through the blood, sweat, and tears with me. Jennifer Martin, I love you for hanging in there with me to the end. Thank you for being there through it all—the sleepless nights, crazy shoots, and being able to speak and translate "Taylor." Margaret Pleyn, thank you for your generous help and for being there through the chaos and for helping me make it happen. I love you dearly. To Carlos Ortiz, thank you for your genius and being so generous with your time.

To Hasblady Guzman and everyone of the Renaissance Family who I grew up with. For letting me play with your faces, giving me my first kit, and for teaching me and supporting me. To Babs and my long-lost sisters Djuna Smith and Jeannie Chea and family, for being there for me when I needed it most. To Kita Huynh, thank you for all of your help during this time; it was priceless. I feel truly blessed to have you all as friends.

All my love to my family, the Changs and Babaians, for your never-ending support, especially Angel, Arshavir, Max, and Jina, thank you for being the first face I got to play with; my husband, Raffi, for helping me in every way to make this book possible; and my incredible children, Adina and Christopher, for their sacrifices and support. To my mother, Anne, thank you for teaching me the meaning of ambition and hard work.

All my gratitude to Laurent Vernhes and Blake Edwards Barnett at Tablet Hotels (www.tablethotels.com). You so get me and my taste. Bonnie Heller at Bryant Park Hotel in New York. Thank you to Richard Morris at Morgans Hotel Group in Miami. NightSnow Vogt at the Clift Hotel in San Francisco and Scott Kawasaki at Hyatt Regency Waikiki.

Maholo to everyone at the FX Group for everything! (www.fx-group.com)

Special thanks to Eduardo Lucero, Elyssa B., Monique Lhullier, Laura Long, and Adele Mildred, for your beautiful designs and support.

Thank you to everyone at Quixote Studios especially Abe Swaidan. Thank you to everyone at 5th and Sunset Studios L.A.; Keith Vallot and my dear friend Elaine Lee; Sasie in San Francisco; my fierce legal support, Ara Babaian. Shant Melkonian, thanks for all of your help throughout the years. Special thanks to my friends in Miami, Gigi and Patrick Salisbury, Frank Navarro, and Jason Louis Zabaleta, for their time and generous contributions. To my friends, Brian Inatsuka and Miguel Soltero, thank you for everything!

Many thanks to everyone who contributed their time and artistic genius to this project. Tiffany Caliva, you believed in it from the beginning. Thank you! Peter Brown, Jim Malucci, Mike Ruiz, Jon McKee, Mitch Stone, Peter Z. Jones, Joe Hill, Rob Latour, Mark Hanauer, Christian Bier-Gross, Will Carrillo, Manuel Benevides, Christine Nguyen, Rondi Ballard, Alfelino Feliciano, Brad Coker, John Shin, and Jerry Riboli.

To Albert Sanchez and Pedro Zalba, thank you for your tireless dedication and generosity to this project and for going beyond the call of duty and really taking this book to the next level.

Special thanks to Amanda Keeley, Amy Zvi, and Cullen Conly. To Elke Von Freudenberg, for telling me that I needed to be a makeup artist all those years ago. I've had the greatest time ever since that day. Lisa Botts and Annie McCullough, for all of her kind words of encouragement throughout the years. Dr. Balfour and team. St. Joseph's Medical Hospital and Wellspring Therapy, you really got me through a tough time and pulled me through. Onnig Sayadian at tsapros.com for all of his tech support.

To Pamela Skaist-Levy and Gela Nash-Taylor, thank you for all your advice and continued support and for inspiring me in so many ways. To Kelly Lebrock, thank you so much for your support and all of your uplifting words.

To all the models, professional and "real" women, THANK YOU for lending me your beautiful faces. All of you are so beautiful inside and out. You have made this little girl's dream come true. Heartfelt gratitude to Charlotte Halford at Wilhelmina, Francine Champagne and Victor at Vision Los Angeles, Mamie Indig at L.A. Models, Cindy Kauanui at Jetset Models, Kenya Knight at Nous Models, Jackie Salem at Elite Models, Shelly Kolsrud at Qmodels, Linda Solis and Jennifer Powell at Next Model Management, George Speros at NY Models, and Jeff at Look.

ALBERT SANCHEZ is a Southern California native. He studied photo-realist painting at Cal State Fullerton, which led to an interest in photography. His career in photography began in Paris as a portrait photographer and expanded into the fields of celebrity portraiture, beauty, and fashion. His photographic style references Hollywood glamour photography and brings it into today's aesthetic. He has worked for a wide variety of entertainment publications, advertising agencies, and record companies. His celebrity portraits include Nicole Kidman, Mick Jagger, Kate Winslet, and Jennifer Lopez. He has shot beauty campaigns for Revlon, L'Oréal, Paul Mitchell, and Wella. Albert enjoys being hands-on in the digital imaging of his photography. His photos appear on pages ii, iv, 16, 46, 50, 54, 66, 102, 116, 132, 136, 138, 140, 144, 150, 156, and 158.

PETER BROWN has enjoyed photographing hundreds of beautiful people from Naomi Cambell, Charlize Theron, and Pink to Paris Hilton, Pete Burns, and even the Pope...He has worked on magazines from *The Face* to British *Vogue*, *Cosmo*, *Maxim*, and many others. He has traveled the world and worked on four continents. Peter hails from London, England, but has called L.A. home for the past ten years. Peter considers himself a lucky man! See his photos on pages 32, 33, 76, 78, 110, 112, 126, and 146.

JON MCKEE was one of the photographers who I started with. His work spans fashion, celebrity, and advertising, and I've been fortunate to have worked on all of the above with him. Jon has a youthful soul that approaches photography with such inspiring excitement. Jon is based in Los Angeles. Visit www.jonmckeephotography.com. Jon's photos appear on pages 36, 64, 74, 82, 88, 94, 100, 104, 106, and 108.

ROB LATOUR, born and raised in Canada, began his professional career teaching mathematics, physics, and chemistry. For Rob, photography provided the needed creative balance he needed. Rob moved to L.A. in 1980 and has photographed celebrities, including Jimmy Stewart, Mary Martin, Jack Lemmon, Julie Andrews, Edward James Olmos, David Hyde Pierce, Linda Evans, Debbie Allen, Kristi Yamaguchi, Giorgio Armani, Tommy Hilfiger, and Van Morrison. See his photos on pages 59, 70, and 92.

JOE HILL has been shooting for more than twenty years and has traveled a good chunk of the world. Joe credits his craft to spending six years living in Europe where he learned who he is today as a photographer. He has shot with magazine giants *Vogue*, *Cosmopolitan*, *Worldwide*, *Vogue Homme*, *Mademoiselle*, *Harper's Bazaar*, and *Brides*. See Joe's on pages 114, 128, 134, 142, and 148.

MIKE RUIZ, a New York-based photographer, is best known for his high-impact, colorful celebrity photography like Beyoncé and Britney Spears as well as his glossy fashion editorials. He frequently shoots the hottest new stars for major American and international magazines including *Vanity Fair*, *Flaunt*, *Interview*, *Latina*, and *Paper*, and was a contributor to Dolce and Gabbana's *Hollywood* book and Iman's *The Beauty of Color* beauty book. His work has also appeared in several European magazines including Italian *Elle*, *Arena*, and *Dazed and Confused*. Mike has shot advertising campaigns for Sean John, MAC Cosmetics, and Candies. Mike has worked with music giants Arista, Badboy Records, RCA, Interscope, TommyBoy Records, EMI, Universal, Sony, TVT, Warner Bros. Records, and Bravo, UPN, USA and SciFi television networks. He has recently branched out as a director, creating music videos for Traci Lords and Kristine W. See Mike's photos on pages 1, 80, 124, and 154.

MITCH STONE originally found himself working in the movie and fashion industry as a hairstylist in Hollywood, working with many of the industry's top stars. From there, he moved to New York City to work with the world's top photographers, designers, models, publications, and campaigns. Working with such photographers as Herb Ritts, Albert Watson, Arthur Elgort, and Peter Arnell, he was able to see their work as an inspiration that refueled his love for the craft of photography. In 1996 he moved back to L.A. to enroll in Santa Monica College School of Photography. Since then, Stone has been requested to shoot celebrity portraits (some of them former hair clients!) and with his background being hair and beauty, he has most recently been shooting campaigns for hair and skin care companies that trust his trained eye. He was recently commissioned by the Tahitian Islands to capture the brilliance of their native black pearls on Marlon Brando's private island. While there, Jean Paul Gaultier saw Mitch's work and, impressed, hired him to capture his runway show. His photos appear on pages 2, 3, 40, 84, 86, 118, 152, and 160.

JIM MALUCCI is a mysterious man of few words and humbly didn't want to give a bio; however, his photos speak for themselves. I met Jim on a celebrity fashion cover shoot and worked with him over a few days on location and was very impressed. He was gracious enough to lend me his talents to shoot the Miami spread (pages 122–123 as well as page 166) and I feel truly blessed to have had him and his crew a part of it.

MICHAEL WILLIAMS, a Canadian-born photographer, jump-started his career in Paris. Michael's work has appeared in international editions of *Vogue, Marie Claire, Elle*, and *GQ*, as well as many independent magazines such as *Arena, Surface*, and *Flaunt*. His advertising credits include FCUK, AX Armani, L'Oréal, and McDonald's. Recent work includes editorials for French *Glamour* and British *GQ*. He has also photographed many celebrities, as well as top models such as Heidi Klum, Naomi Campbell, Carolyn Murphy, and Angela Lindvall. Michael is well-known for his professional ease on set, his quickness, and an intuitive understanding of his clients' needs. Quickly becoming one of the world's finest beauty photographers, he is also renowned for shooting fashion and personalities. Michael resides in New York City and divides his time between the United States and Europe. See his photos on page 72.

MARK HANAUER, a native Californian, has been creating images for the advertising, entertainment, editorial, and athletic industries for several years. Mark was the chief photographer for A&M Records. He has taught at the Art Center College of Design. Past clients include Nike, Adidas, Condé Nast Publications, Paramount, Sony, and Quiksilver. Mark is represented by JG+A (www.jgaonline.com). See his photos on pages 15, 68, 96, and 98.

JENNIFER MARTIN has loved fashion since she was a little girl and started early on in the fashion industry styling for some of the biggest department stores in America. Her strong work ethic and fun-loving personality has allowed her to work with some of the industry's best artists and photographers. Jennifer is the lead stylist for *Asian Faces* and lives in Los Angeles with her husband, Frank, and children, Ashley and Jason.

San Francisco (page 130) photographed by Peter Z. Jones.
Product photos by John Shin, Rob Latour, and Jerry Riboli.
Photo of Yoko Ono and the author by Amanda Keeley.
Yunjin Kim styled by Erin Turon.
Margaret Cho styled by Clint Catalyst and Geisha Fumi Akutagawa.

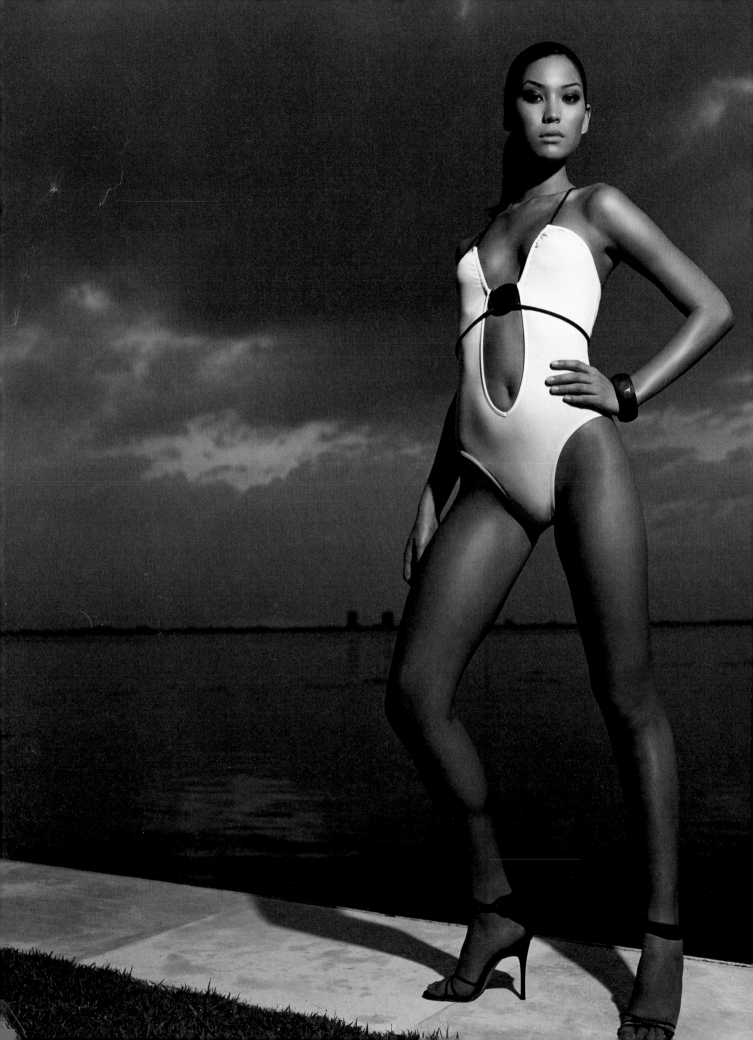